GUIDED MEDITATION FOR DEEP SLEEP

GUIDED MEDITATION FOR DEEP SLEEP: RELAXATION AND STRESS RELIEF. HELPS YOU TO FALL ASLEEP FASTER, REDUCE ANXIETY, STOP DEPRESSION, AND NEGATIVE THINKING. MINDFULNESS MEDITATION TO WAKE UP HAPPY.

Table of Contents

Introduction

Sit somewhere where you are able to entirely relax. Don't choose a spot where there is a high level of distraction. This can be done in a group, but it is only suggested as long as everyone is entirely dedicated to the meditation. You will get the best results when you can do this in solitude. When picking a location to do this, ensure that it is one filled with positive energy. You don't want to select a location that is in a high traffic area. This could affect the flow of energy as it passes through you.

Start to focus on your breathing. Allow the air to come in and out of your body naturally. Pay attention to the way that the air fills you up and how it flows so freely out after your body has done all the work of recycling it. Breathe in and out. In and out.

We are going to count down from twenty. It is suggested that you are breathing in through your nose and out through your mouth as this is going to give you the best pattern of regulated breathing. Breathe in through your nose and out through your mouth for five seconds each time.

Breathe in for one, two, three, four, and five, and out for five, four, three, two, and one.

Continue this pattern as you travel throughout this meditation. We are going to take you on a journey through your body in the spiritual plane. Close your eyes and choose a position where you are not blocking any flow through your body. If you choose to sit up straight in a cross-legged position, that's perfectly fine. For beginners it is OK to choose a position where you are stretched out and totally relaxed. We are going to count down from twenty. When we reach one, the meditation will begin.

You have seven chakras that exist inside of you. They start at the base of your spine and work their way all the way up to the top of your head. Many individuals will go throughout their entire lives without tapping in to the chakras. When one of your chakras is blocked, then it will affect every other one. It is a flow and a passage through your body, so it is important that we keep everything in harmony working with each other, rather than against each other.

Chapter 1 What Is Sleep Meditation?

You might wonder what sleep meditation is. I mean, how can you meditate while you sleep? Well, there is a certain way to utilize this, and a various set of factors that go into this, and in this chapter, we'll discuss just what sleep meditation entails.

Now, often when people are stressed, they use meditation when they are trying to calm their nerves. Well, when you're sleeping, you can't exactly sit there and tell yourself to not do something, or just completely be there? It's kind of hard to sleep in the lotus position, right? Well, sleep meditation gives you the factors necessary in order to engage in meditation all while you fall asleep.

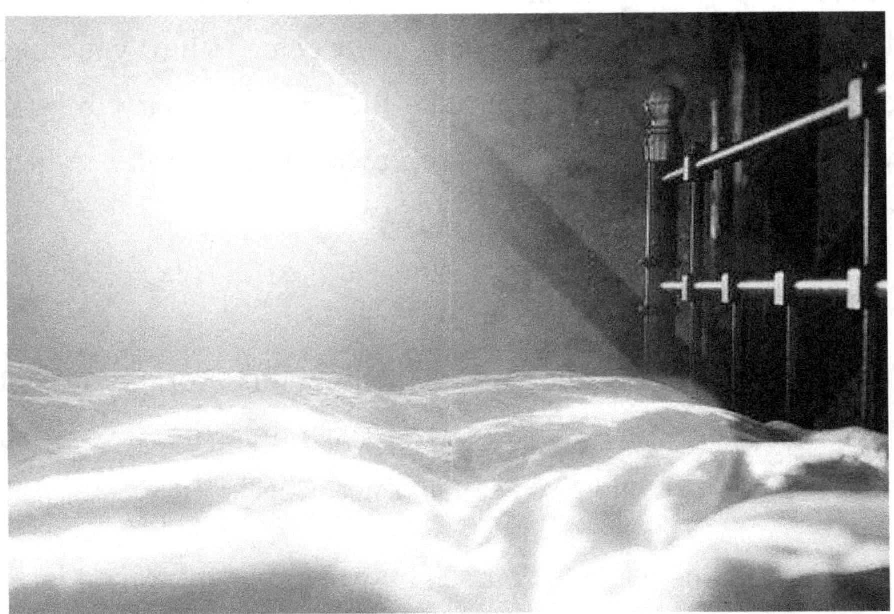

It's a natural way to help calm the body down, relax the muscles, and give you better sleep.

Lots of us have very overactive minds that are filled with stress and other factors that only make us feel worse when we get up. If you don't sleep, you'll end up hurting yourself, and this form of meditation gives you a means to sleep better, feel better, and to live a better life.

Meditate is a great way to find out more about your body, to become more mindful of various actions that might be going on there, and to help you build a better, more remunerative existence. Your sleep schedule, and how much you sleep, does affect the going ons in the mind and in what you do in real life the next day as well. You need to be focused on what you do during the day, since often you're working, making money, or the like. Being asleep during the day is only going to hurt you more and more, so it's best if you take the time necessary to relax yourself, your body, and use sleep meditation in order to help you better your life.

Meditation For Quick Rest

When you are in the middle of something, like work, or a tight schedule, you might need to give yourself a short time so you can have a quick rest, and also get your energy back.

You can use this script to yourself how to have a quick rest in 10 minutes

- Sit in a comfortable position you may not need to change your chair or location, except you are in a distracting environment

- Close your eyes at your own convenient time,

- Feel the sensation of your eyes been closed, feel the state of your eyes resting

- The sensation that comes from the resting of your closed eyelids, and let them get softened and rest more

- Allow them to soften on their own, and begin to feel rest in your mind

- Let your eyes know they only need to rest, instead of working hard and staring at some objects because they are opened. By letting your eyes know this, you are giving them permission to be in this restful state.

- As your eyes are getting more soften, engage yourself with the softening and enjoy this sensation of resting your eyes, and not having them doing anything

- At this point, focus your attention on your mind

- In your own convenient time, allow your mind to feel the same thing your eyes is feeling right now. Let your mind soften

- Sit back in your head and feel as your mind is becoming softened.

- Let your mind know it does not have to work or do anything right now. Your mind does not need to worry about anything or feel anxious.

- You also need to give your mind permission to rest.

- Allow your mind to engage well with this rest, and sit back and feel the sensation coming from this softening

- You also need to allow any sense of importance on your mind to soften

- As long as you are enjoying this sensation, allow your mind to soften and move towards resting on its own

- Focus your awareness on your physical body, not looking down at your body, but paying attention, and sensing into your physical body's weight, and contact the physical body's making with the support beneath you.

- Let your physical body soften and really feel comfortable in the support

- Give your physical body the permission to rest, let it know it does not need to do anything.

- Allow your body to soften, and let this softening spread across your body parts, gently bringing your awareness through your body

- You also focus your attention on your body parts, by allowing these pars to soften and rest. You can start with your shoulders, let your shoulders become flat, and then softening and rest your shoulders

- You are giving them permission to your arms, to get softened and also get into a state of rest

- You are allowing your body to soften, and rest

- All your body parts are softening, and resting on the support beneath you

- And as your mind, and the body sits back into the support beneath them. Allow your breath to soften, and allow your breath to release all that healthy breath, and also give it the permission to breathe in a certain way.

- Let your breath be free, let it soften, and at the end flow on its own term.

- As you move towards rest, and as your breath softens and slows down, draw any part of u, perhaps you back, and thigh, that has always uncomfortable either in the present of past, let them soften and sit back to be supported by the present sensation.

- Do not forget to give all of your permission to your body parts to rest, your mind, back, face. Every part of you should be given permission to rest.

- Begin to have an awareness of what happens when you soften and allow yourself to rest, and in your own time, you can conclude this meditation.

- You can open your eyes when you are ready, still sitting back with your mind, body, and eyes soft.

- As you put an end to this meditation, enjoy this restful state as you return to your work.

After Work Relieving Stress Meditation

Guided De-Stressing Mantra

With this short guide, you can easily de-stress yourself from feeling stressed out, overwhelmed and also tired.

- Sit in a comfortable position

- Take a deep breath first, then hold your breath, take a pause, and take a few deep breaths right now

- Make sure you breathe in deeply and notice that as you breathe in, you feel the air going into your abdomen, as your abdomen is rising more than your chest is rising.

- Spend enough time, perhaps a few seconds to notice how you are feeling. You may notice you are feeling overwhelmed, pressure from work, or feeling unsatisfied as you are reflecting on all that happened during the day.

- You can spend a few seconds affirming how you want to feel at the end of this meditation.

  'I am feeling stressed right now, but I am beginning to get de-stressed'

'I was angry at work today, but I am beginning to feel good and happy'

'I am not feeling crossed at anyone, not even my boss or myself'

- It is okay that you felt stressed, and tired at work, but you are beginning to feel very relieved as you let go of these negative feelings.

- Take a deep breath at work, and imagine that your worries and stresses are going down the drain

- Imagine you are at the water basin, and you open the tap, and as the tap stats running, you feel your stress and worries are going down the drain

- As you begin to feel this relieve in your mind, you should create a supportive and positive environment for this feeling

- You will begin to say positive words about yourself, work and relationship.

'I am the best staff in my company'

'I have a positive and good customer care'

'I am wise in decision making'

'I make good friends both in my office and outside my office'

'I am loved by other staff of my company, my boss inclusive'

'I create good solutions and I am creative'

'I am perfect, and I do not give anybody the permission to make me feel bad and inferior'

- How do you feel saying those positive affirmations?

- Take a pause, still with your eyes closed. Take a deep breath in and out

- Then take another breathe, this time slowly as you begin to feel your worries and stress fade away

- As you enjoy this sensation, shift your focus and pay more attention to your mind.

- You are beginning to feel more confident as you are becoming de-stressed.

- You take another deep breath and breathe out slowly.

- You are feeling much relieved and happy. As you continue breathing, you are letting go of everything and you are becoming more relieved and confident.

Guided Meditation For Calmness

When you are stressed, you are always overwhelmed and you will need to be calm. This guided script will make you achieve calmness in a short minute.

- Sit in a comfortable position, as I invite you to this relieving meditation to regain calmness

- As you feel settled into this calm atmosphere, take a deep breath, hold your breath and breathe out.

- Close your eyes as soon as you want to get into this calm atmosphere

- Imagine what it feels like to be calm; if calmness has a color, what color did you think it will be?

- If calmness had a scent, what scent will it be?

- Begin to let your mind sink into what it feels like to be calm.

- Take a deep breath and pause

- You are taking a pause because you need to know it feels to be calm, what it means for your mind to be calm

- Then focus on your mind, and pay attention to the worries of your mind. You can still hear the troubles and worries of your mind; you can still hear the voice of your last client complaining and yelling at you. You can still see the look on your competitor's face at the pitching event.

- You can still see yourself scared of the unknown

- Now, take a deep breath and let all these worries go down to the earth beneath your feet, as you hold your breath. You can breathe out now

- Imagine what it feels like you to have a good client who will always be satisfied with your services or a good team that is loving and hardworking

- You begin to feel your mind calm, and all your worries are gone

- Imagine you are in front of a whiteboard, with a marker in your hands.

- Write down your worries and struggles, as you feel more calm

- As you are writing them, you are erasing them, and you feel more calm

- You feel relieved, as there are no struggles around you anymore

- How do you feel now? Take a deep breath in and out.

- Smile widely as you feel calmer than ever.

- You can open your eyes when you need to. You can also repeat the exercise when you want to feel calm.

Relieving Stress Hypnosis

You are about to get into a hypnotic state, where your consciousness will be quiet.

- Get into a comfortable position, you can choose to sit down or lie down.

- Close your eyes and let your focus be on your mind

- Breath in and out

- As you breathe in, you see your mind becoming relieved, no more stress or struggles. You are becoming safe within your self

- Imagine you are at the entrance of a beautiful room, with the title tag 'solution room.'

- You walk into this room, and all you see is darkness, with a little light ray on a chair and table

- You sit on this chair and feel a different sensation

- You cannot explain this sensation, but you feel better, and great feeling relieved and stresses

- The ray of light is still shining on you, and you are beginning to see more clearly than you first entered the room.

- Take deep breathe in and out and lift your head to the ceiling

- You begin to count the number of boxes you can see on the ceiling, the more you count, and the more your eyes are becoming heavy and sleepy.

- You feel your eyelids heavier and sleepier, and it looks like it wants to fall off

- You stop counting the ceiling now, and you feel more relaxed and better

- You are very relieved and relieved as you feel take another deep breath

- You are getting deep into relieve and deeper into sleeping

- Feel more comfortable in this state, and enjoy this sensation of this state.

- You can stand up from this chair, and walk towards the entrance of the door

- You open the door and come out of this dark room

- As you are out of the room, all your worries are gone and disappeared

- Take a deep breath in and out

- Enjoy this moment and feel relieved

- Begin to get back into your body, and feel this sensation

- You still have your eyes closed. You feel deeply relieved and calm

- You can open your eyes now, and enjoy the feeling

- How do you feel now?

- Feel how relieved you are right now

Visual Meditation For Stress

- Get into a comfortable position

- Take a deep breath in and out

- Open your mouth and breathe in through your mouth, as you breathe out through your nose

- Take another breath slowly, and this time close your eyes slightly

- You are about to get into a relaxed state, and you are about to deal with stress

- Think of your struggles at work, and visualize them

- You do not need to imagine anything right now, just visualize the problems you face at work. Like your bills, your next presentation, your proposal, and the next interview.

- As you visualize these problems, take a deep breath in and out.

- I want you to see how your problems look, and see them fading away.

- As they fading away, you begin to feel relieved, and calm

- Breathe in slowly, and breathe out through your nose.

- Imagine that you are floating up in the clouds, and as the clouds are moving you are getting relaxed and comfortable

- You do not need to know where the cloud is taking you to, just calm down and enjoy this moment

- Inhale the fresh air from the sky, and exhale the air through your mouth

- The cloud is drawing closer to your office, and soon you are floating above the roof of your office.

- You feel calm and relieved even as the cloud lowers you to the ground and as you get down to feel the earth beneath you

- You feel the earth beneath you is becoming soft, as you feel like sinking into the ground

- You feel comfortable walking on the ground, as you keep walking your office

- Now that you are in your workplace, imagine that there is an elevator. You get into this elevator, and as this elevator goes upward, you feel relieved. The more relieved you feel, the calmer you are.

- In this elevator, you feel you are in a different world entirely. You feel this sensation, even more as you enjoy this moment

- The elevator is in front of the board room, and as you walk out of the elevator, you feel the ground soft, and you feel like sinking into it

- You walk on the ground comfortably and walk into the board room

- Imagine the board room is dark, with nobody in there

- As soon as you take a seat, the light comes on, and you feel even more calm and relieved

- In this board room, you begin to hear a solemn song playing. You feel calm, and relieved

- You begin to let go of the awkward and overwhelming feeling you got from the last board meeting. As you breathe in slowly and hold your breath, you let go of the resentment you have towards your colleagues at work.

- You feel good and cozy as you let go of these issues, like anger, disappointments, and struggles.

- Take another deep breath in and out, and enjoy the song playing in the background

- You are feeling calm, and relieved

- Now, shift your attention towards your mind. Search inwards your body and mind, and find the intentions of your heart. You begin to see the fears you have towards your next project

- Take a deep breath in and out

- Stand up from your seat and walk around the board table. As you walk around, you feel calmer and comfortable

- In this room, there are 12 chairs, and you begin to count each chair and touch them.

- You touch the first chair and count. As you count, you become calmer and more relieved. Then you touch other chairs, from the second to the fifth chair, to the eighth chair. You realized you are calmer as you count more numbers.

- You count the last number, 12 and you feel like a load was lifted off you. You return to your seat and sit calmly

- Your eyes are feeling heavy, so you rest your head on the table to catch some sleep. You are about dozing off, but you are awake because you feel a cold hand patting your shoulder.

- You look up and see the man looking at you and smiling. He says hello and welcomes you to his world.

- You look around and wonder what he means, he tells you not to be afraid but rather trust in what he has to say to you.

- He asks you to take a deep breath in and out, he then asks you to rest your back comfortably on the chair.

- As you sit comfortably, he asks you to focus on your mind, and say out the first issues your mind brings to you. You close your eyes and do as he said; the first thing your mind brings up is about your relationship with your boss.

- You feel calm about the selection, and you are beginning to drift into a sleepy state.

- The man snaps his finger and you wake up.

- He tells you to write in a paper what 5 things you like about your boss and 5 things you dislike about him. He also asks you to write 5 ways you can help your boss become better.

- As you write this, you become calmer, you are smiling and you are beginning to imagine yourself and your boss having a long and interesting conversation the next day.

- You write it all, and the man asks you to keep it. He smiles at you again and walks out of the room.

- You are feeling unusual, and good about this, but you are stuck in the conference room

- You walk out since feeling relaxed and calm; you get into the elevator to take you downstairs. As you go down, you are beginning to have slight control over your environment, but not fully

- You imagine you are floating back in the sky. You are returning home, and you still feel the sensation coming from calmness.

- You are in your bed now, you feel great, and your mind is settled. You have the solutions to your problems, and you feel slightly awake and conscious right now

- You can begin to open your eyes gradually and return back to your normal activities

- You are fully awake and refreshed, now you can go back to work.

This meditation is an example; you can write your scripts anyhow you want. You can also choose whatever meditation technique that goes well with.

Chapter 2 Pre-Meditation: Preparing To Drop In

To ensure that you have a successful meditation free of distractions, there are some things you may want to incorporate in the hours before you crawl into bed. Setting the stage for a night of deep rest may involve getting rid of some old habits and allowing some new changes in your bedtime routine. Some of these may seem obvious, will put an end to your insomnia fast. It may be one lousy habit of keeping you from getting the rest that you need. To ready the mind and body for bed, try incorporating some of the following tips.

Make sure you complete any task that may keep your mind up at night. If preparing stuff for the next day would help, do so settling in. If you have tasks that need to wait until tomorrow, acknowledge them and write them down. Putting down all your tasks on a list will help your mind let go of them for the time being. After writing them down detach from them and know you can think about it in the morning. Often the most significant source of our sleepless nights is based on the overwhelming to-do list for tomorrow. Even though it is natural to run through all these things before rest, it is actually inhibiting you from achieving a relaxed state of mind, and it is revving up all those anxiety-inducing, task-based beta brainwaves. It will be a lot more of a challenge to dive into the meditative process fully if you are unable to let go of all the things that are needed to be done. Meditation is about being right here and now at the moment, so the past and future will do its best to take you out of it.

Consider starting a nightly journaling practice to help settle all the mental chatter from the day. If things happened during the last day or week that have you ruminating and running through them at night, journaling would help sort them out. The act of writing down all your thoughts, problems, and relationship difficulties helps you to take a step away from them and really decide what is worth all the emotional energy. You will often find that much of what you fixate on in the mind is absolute rubbish. Your brain thinks and analyzes so much it will go over the top so you will end up putting way more weight to things and problems than needed. Most of the thoughts in the brain are pointless, and it is possible that you will get stuck in a mental loop going back over again things that do not need revisiting. Journaling will help you through processing all the thoughts and happenings at the end of the day. It will feel much easier turning off the brain when you set free some of the pressing and unhelpful thought patterns.

Take a good hard look at the kinds of habits you are currently doing before bed. If you go to bed whenever you feel like, try to stick with a set and regular bedtime every night to train your internal clock. When you go to bed sporadically, your body is not always prepared to rest. When you have a set time every night that you go to sleep, your body knows and expects it. It will grow tired closer to that set time, and by listening and becoming more in tune with your body, you can know and be ready for rest as well. Make sure that the environment you fall asleep in is warm and comfortable. Abstain from doing anything in your bed other than sleeping or having sex. Do not use your bed for work, eating, or watching TV. Even though it is enjoyable to do these things in the comfort of your own bed, you train yourself subconsciously that it is a place where you can be awake and doing things. When you use your bed only for resting the brain will take note and become more relaxed when you are ready to ease down under the covers.

The things you do before the meditation can help or hinder the success of it depending on what they are. If you are the type of person that loves staring at their phone until they are ready to try and sleep, consider changing your ways. The blue light from phones or any electronic suppresses the production of melatonin. Melatonin is the sleep-inducing hormone that regulates your body's internal clock. When you are not producing melatonin as regularly as needed, you will find it harder to fall asleep and get quality hours of rest. Two hours before bed should be blue light free to help the brain produce the chemicals needed for sleep. Activities and habits before bed should be comfortable and stimulant-free.

Avoid caffeine in the later afternoon and evening. Even if you do not feel the full effects, it still will give you a slightly wired mental energy. Also, if you think the caffeine will wear off shortly know that it has a half-life of 3-5 hours, with the remainder hanging around in your system even longer. It takes even longer to process if you are an older adult. Its stimulating effects will make it harder to fall asleep, and studies have shown that it delays the timing on your internal clock. Caffeine can be the sole cause of your insomnia, and you may not even be aware that it is keeping you up. If you drink any caffeinated beverages in the latter part of the day, try experimenting and put them down for the time being. You may notice a big difference with the amount of time it takes to fall asleep.

Other things to avoid if you want a better night's sleep are alcohol and nicotine. Nicotine also acts in a stimulating manner and may rev up your system before rest. While alcohol can make it easier to drift off, it will not let you reach deeper stages of sleep and will wake you up earlier than intended. Drinking will leave you feeling drained and dehydrated in the morning and eating too much before bed can make it hard to get comfortable and come with side effects like heartburn and bad digestion. It is best to stay away from these sorts of vices that will hurt your health and sleep. Drinking a warm cup of herbal tea such as chamomile or lavender can be a good switch. Tea has positive, relaxing properties to it and will aid you in getting a better night's rest.

Stretching out the muscles and joints and breathing is an excellent thing to consider doing before you begin your meditation. Yoga, the art of breathing and stretching has been used throughout time to prepare the body for a still seated meditation. By moving around and breathing, you release any trapped tightness and tension. Yoga and meditation go hand in hand to bring balance, peace, and relaxation to the body. By incorporating a simple yoga practice into your life, and before bed, you can get even faster results in the amount of rest you have.

Simple stretches could be raising and pulling the arms overhead or folding forward over the legs. When doing yoga at night before bedtime, it is best to do poses that are gentler with longer holds. Folding forward and grabbing onto opposite elbows, you can stay here for a good few minutes watching the breath and noticing how the body feels in this position. A position that greatly reduces your blood pressure and stress is putting your legs up a wall. All you have to do is press your buttocks into a supporting wall, swing the legs up and over and sit. Take long, deep breaths while in this position and feel all the stagnant blood flow down out of your legs and into your heart. Hold this position for at least five minutes allowing the legs to go numb. When you have had enough, ease out slowly, and rest on the floor for a few minutes allowing recirculation to happen through the legs.

It is all about leaving the doing behind before bedtime, so limit things that require too much stimulation. Even vigorous exercise right before bed can get your energy going too strong. Keep everything light and simple and relaxed, allowing your mind to unwind from a busy day. Creating healthy habits at night can be a good basis for a restful meditation practice and serve you in easing your insomnia. Employing some of these added solutions will get you on the road to sleeping better sooner.

Chapter 3 The Importance Of Meditation

The use of meditation has already been approved psychologically to be useful and helpful. It assists the human body to cope with depression. Depression hurts everyone's life despite their age. It is almost impossible to deny and snob the merits of meditation to the human body and mind. Once the mind is disturbed and unsettled, this is where meditation comes in to help calm and connect the two. When this happens, the soul of the person meditating is raised to a higher consciousness hence leading to being more aware. Being aware of one's self helps in the accumulation of universal knowledge, which is power. This chapter will be dealing with the physiological and psychological benefits of meditation. The merits of meditation play a significant role in one's success, and they are as follows:

Attention to the psychological benefits of meditation has grown. The psychological benefits of meditation assist the mind of the person practicing meditation. Activities involved in meditation are mental. We are in a world that is continuously evolving to new things. As technology advances, new medications continue to emerge. Some people want a happy life without these medications. They rely on the holistic and natural healing power of meditation. New and old natural forms of meditation are acquiring positive criticism.

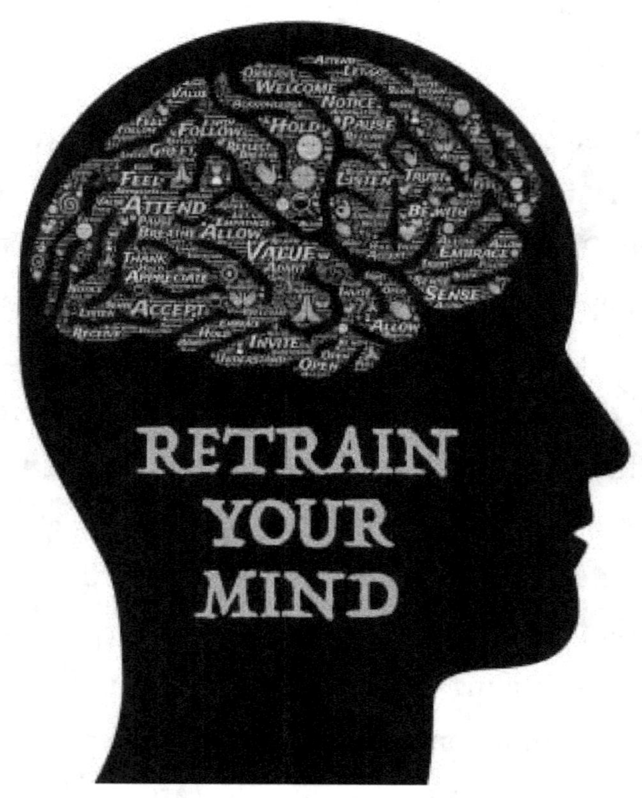

Meditation Relieves Stress

Since meditation has gained popularity within the human civilization, it remains to be the number of stress reliever in the world. People who tend to meditate daily have an almost zero percent life stress and are thriving. Fear has been one of the top health issues in the world. The number of adults reporting stress problems is increasing by a staggering percentage within the past few years. Life has a lot of difficulties and challenges. The struggles and hustling of modern life have become a way of life. Stress is part of life that makes it interesting. Stress in small quantities can enhance people to perform better under pressure.

Science says that stress can alter and change the brain physiology.

You can define stress as "being a response from the body or mind to a particular demand." The effect depends on the intensity, time, and remedy used. Stress starts when the brain sends a signal to the hypothalamus; once this happens, it leads to the secretion of cortisol "the stress hormone." This hormone in large quantities can shrink the brain and hence lowering the brain's normal functioning. The conditions and environment that trigger stress is called stressors. Most people view stress as a negative thing. However, any experience or situation that puts pressure on us is stressful. Some of them include getting a raise as promotion, acquiring mortgages, or joining college. Some stress we tend to generate it ourselves. Being too occupied, perfectionism, or expecting things that are not achievable can cause anxiety. The worst thing that stress can do to us is that it can hold on to us to the extent that we get used to it.

A stressed-out person exhibits signs and symptoms. Most of the signs are cognitive. Meditation comes in handy when a person is under stress. The type of meditation that can curb this kind of situation you can call it mindfulness meditation. Research on grownups has shown that mindfulness meditation can decrease the amount of stress that an individual experiences. Its effectiveness is maximum for people who experience stress most and meditate on a daily routine. Once the depression is relieved, a persons' wellbeing grows. It also leads to the reduction of stress-related issues like fibromyalgia and post-traumatic stress disorder. A life with a prolonged stress period can change the brain's neural connections. It makes us more vulnerable to other stress stimuli. If not maintained, stress can lead to other related problems, such as autoimmune diseases. Every person has a different ability to deal with stress. Some can strive in a Stressful situation, while others will be frustrated.

Healing Depression and Anxiety

You can define a healthy mind as one with no mental disorder. Mental health these days can be improved. These improvements can be made in various ways. The leading one is meditation. Meditation is both an individual and spiritual experience. Anxiety is an emotion associated with worry and tension. Everyone feels stress. Anxiety affects everyone. Here we will go through with dealing with it. Most people do not understand it. It is not just a feeling. Anxiety can never fade away. Regardless of where you are, you will always feel it. Through meditative inhalation and exhalation daily. One can improve his or her ability to deal with anxiety. Anxiety can prevent a person from working at full potential. Stress can lead to high blood pressure. This happens when it is not maintained. It can also induce restlessness. It can also cause worry, which is uncontrollable. Anxiety can also hinder one from sleeping. Stress can lead to anger.

Meditation can help reduce anxiety. People who suffer from anxiety can overcome it. By using mindfulness meditation, one can minimize anxiety efficiently.

People think that their life is complete. No. Fear pops up. Have a huge event coming. Most of the cases of anxiety are unexpected. Meditation is the cheapest way to deal with stress. It is more effective than drugs. Its effects are long-lasting. When compared to drugs, it is more affordable and more effective. This therapy is very successful in treating depression and anxiety. These effects are long-term. The method is also less costly. Just after a few months into the program, some of the patients were already well. So, meditation works better than antidepressants to reduce anxiety. The world is full of chaos. Chaos can exert some stress in you. However, with a peaceful mind, we can deal with the disorder. Therefore, this is where peace in the brain is required.

You can eventually achieve this through meditation.

Meditation can also be used with antidepressants. Mindfulness meditation assists a lot in this sector. To reduce anxiety, one meditates by focusing on the heart. Fortunately, it boosts confidence within the meditator. With this, the more stable a person will become. One imagines that the soul is breathing. The breathing should be sincere. The person meditating should also add a feeling of appreciation. This should be practiced frequently as much as possible. During this time, the meditator should think of a he or she is grateful for and highly appreciates — psychology advice people to lean on meditation to reduce anxiety. There are several types of stress. We shall highlight them. We shall look at how to deal with it through meditation.

☐   Generalized anxiety disorder- This induces excess anxiety for an extended period. Unspecified life events cause this anxiety. It is most challenging to identify. This type of stress can be maintained. The remedy for this anxiety is also mindfulness meditation. Addition of an object to concentrate increases efficiency.

☐   Specific phobia- This is the fear that is induced by anxiety. This is triggered by a particular situation. This anxiety is irrational. This is also reduced by mindfulness meditation.

The human brain has many neuron communicators. These communicators are connected. These connections are complex. The communicators are known as "neurotransmitters." There two main neurotransmitters. These are norepinephrine. Every person suffering from depression should be aware of these two. When the level of these two is balanced, we tend to feel good. However, when they are at a low level, we tend to be sad. This leads to us being depressed. Most of the antidepressants taken aim these two neurotransmitters. The issue with antidepressants is that they have unknown side effects. Some of them are addictive. They may not work on some people. Scientific evidence has shown that meditation is ultra-powerful.

A study was done at the University of Montreal by motivated students. They found that meditation can increase neurotransmitters naturally to a healthy level. These are serotonin and norepinephrine. This will bring about a neurochemical utopia. This is a state where depression cannot thrive. The serotonin created as a result of meditation combats all other depression-related issues. A motivated Harvard neuroscientist conducted a study on several meditation practitioners. He later found that the amygdalae of the meditators completely reduced in size. The amygdalae are part of the brain responsible for depression. This part was also less electrically active. In simple terms, meditation switched off the part involved with depression. So, to anyone suffering depression, meditation is the best remedy.

Through meditation, we can be aware of our negative thoughts. These negative thoughts can be a nasty trigger of distress. Meditation prevents this trigger from causing the depression, apart from making us feel mood less. Depression can alter the size and strength of our brains. A study conducted on several depression sufferers. The researchers found out that the hippocampus of the test subjects was so underdeveloped. Hippocampus is the part of the brain known for memory loss and disorientation. They also found, the more a person underwent depression, the more the hippocampus shrank. They then thought of a way to reduce this effect, thus coming up with meditation. Several studies have shown that meditation practitioners tend to have a highly developed and healthy hippocampus — the more years in meditation, the higher hippocampal grey matter density. In simple terms, the more you meditate, the larger and stiff your hippocampus becomes. This causes your brain to rise above all forms of depression.

However, it is not a must for you to practice meditation for several years for you to see the outcomes. Meditation begins to work within days or weeks into meditation. For centuries meditation has been building calmer, focused, and healthier brains. This has been scientifically proven. Every time our minds fire neurons. This produces electrical signals. Once these signals are combined, they form "brainwave patterns." What we are, from our bodies to feelings, introspection is directly measured by brainwave patterns without forgetting depression. Almost thirty years ago, research on depressed alcoholics was done by Biofeedback Institute. This research involved the use of alpha and theta brainwave patterns. The aim was to use these patterns to heal depression. After the therapy, it was found that their depression decreased by eighty percent. Most neuroscientists love studying our brains for lots of reasons. One being, meditation efficiently increases the alpha and theta brainwaves. For example, to acquire these brainwave patterns with ease, one can use the EquiSync.

Meditation has been the secret to having advanced, balanced, and healthy brains. A large amount of evidence has been obtained on the healing power of meditation on depression. This evidence confirms a quick and safe remedy for depression. We, as humans, try to control our emotions. The part of the brain responsible for this is called the "prefrontal cortex." A research done by Pascual-Leone on depressed patients found that this part of their brain was underdeveloped. These patients had a tough time controlling their emotions. Sara Lazar, a Harvard neuroscientist, proved that the minds of meditation practitioners had a developed "prefrontal cortex gray matter." In simple terms, the more time you spend meditating, the more resilient and better your prefrontal cortex becomes. This leads to higher emotional intelligence. This gives you the power to control and manage your emotional life better. Research has shown that meditators are the smartest, have good health, and the happiest among us.

Meditation helps to reduce sleeplessness and insomnia. One of the best sleepers in this world is the people who meditate. If there would be a race to sleep, the meditators will win without a hustle. Here we will be looking at how to use meditation to cure sleeplessness. Sleep is essential as the food we eat. Rest is almost similar to the case of food and the stomach. The human being not only requires sleep but to sleep efficiently.

We depend on sleep for our wellbeing. As human beings, we all have chores. For example, people have to make a living. These activities make us exhausted, and we fatigue. Most of us tend not to get enough sleep. The scientist has been studying our sleeping brains for years. Until recently, they have now understood how it functions. The human brain is one of the big industries in the body. It produces several neurochemicals. One of the influential neurochemicals produced by the brain is melatonin. This is also referred to as the sleep hormone. It is mostly produced just before bedtime. It ensures our body gets a deep and restful sleep. This hormone has its inhibitors. Inhibitors prevent the secretion of this hormone. Stress is one of the inhibitors of melatonin. This inhibits our natural sleep cycle. For us, humans, we are fortunate to have a natural remedy. Researchers at Rutgers University uncovered that meditators had a higher level of melatonin.

Most of the biological markers for sleep are naturally balanced through meditation. This ensures that you get a good night's sleep. The advantages are that the sleep is super deep, and you feel recharged in the morning. This gives no room for insomnia. When we are depressed, our brains tend to have beta brainwaves. The same thing also happens when we are anxious. Beta brainwaves in excess have a detriment effect. Once they are in excess, they can prevent us from sleeping efficiently. This failure to sleep can lead to more productions of beta brainwaves. This is a major complaint from many insomnia patients. This cycle repeats itself to ensure we do not fall asleep. Research shows that meditation practitioners who achieve deep state meditation tend to have a lower attack of insomnia. They also produce fewer beta brainwaves. Instead, they provide more beneficial alpha and theta brainwave patterns. Anyone wanting a good night's sleep should use meditation as his or her remedy.

Most of us tend not to sleep sometimes at night due to the never-ending list of things to do. This is a natural phenomenon.

However, to some extent, it will leave us deprived of sleep, which is not an excellent factor in our lives. These can lower our energy and affect our health in return. Mindfulness meditation teaches us to be aware of the present moment. This awareness also includes our thoughts. This awareness of our body and feelings and how they affect us in the present is the primary way to calm your mind and get sleep. We can use meditation to train our bodies to be ready to sleep.

Meditation Assists in Conquering Addictions

The entire human race happens to have an addiction, whether it is healthy or not healthy at all. Meditation is one of the best methods to overcome an addiction. A study conducted by the American Journal of psychiatry discovered the role of different parts of the brain in addiction. They also found out that the prefrontal cortex or the happiness center becomes active when a person is intoxicated (gets a hit). The same region is underactive when there is a withdrawal. There is a way to activate the prefrontal cortex naturally, and that is through meditation. Sara Lazar conducted a study on the meditator. She found that the neural density and the prefrontal cortex of meditators we highly active. So how does this deal with addiction? Through meditation, we can achieve natural highness. This will be achieved through training of the body and mind to be happy. This highness does not require caffeine or any form of drugs. This good feeling does not lack any addictive substance. Through meditation, we remain to be addiction-free beings — a study done by the American journal of drug and alcohol abuse on patients with drug addiction.

The patients were put through electroencephalogram Biofeedback training; this involves the use of brainwave patterns. This therapy takes the brainwave patterns of the patient to another level of awareness. After twelve months, almost eighty percent of the addicts were drug-free people. The study also showed that in the meditation state, the alpha and beta brainwaves are dominated. This indicates that meditation can be used to treat addiction. It is natural. People suffering from addiction have an urge to satisfy their craving. It is almost overwhelming. This behavior can be self-destructing. With meditation, we can overcome such action. Meditation assists us from being controlled by such things. This method guides the mind from addictive thought. Through meditation, our mind observes without judging the craving and urges as they pass away. When you gain control of your mind through meditation, theurges start reducing. The urges can no longer control you.

Research on the human has been done many addicts. Scientists have discovered a brain chemical called "dopamine." This brain chemical is released into the blood when an addict gets a hit. This chemical is released in specific regions such as "nucleus accumbens." The dopamine levels were found to be low when the addict crushes. This forces him or her to seek more dopamine, hence creating a cycle. The researchers were looking for a way that is natural to counter the dopamine release behavior. A study by John Kennedy showed that dopamine quantities of the addicts were boosted by sixty percent while they were meditating. Their dopamine levels were optimum and in healthy portions. This caused the addicts to avoid crushing.

The University of Washington researched prisoners for ninety days. The inmates were victims of substance addiction. These inmates were put through meditation classes. They performed well in mastering meditation. After ninety days, they were found to consume less of the addictive substance. Those who continued meditating ended up being drug-free. Meditation has been proved to be six times more powerful than any other method to deal with an addiction. This is a perfect example of the healing power of meditation. The number one cause of addiction is sadness. By living a fully aware life, one can never become sad. This full awareness arises from the continuous practice of meditation.

Meditation Maintains Your Focus and Boosts Motivation

Focus and motivation are essential for one's success. In history, people have endured challenges. These challenges never made them give up. A perfect example is Dr. Seuss and his book "Green Egg and Ham." His writing was declined to publish. His book was not only rejected by one publisher but twenty-seven different publishers.

Another example is Oprah Winfrey. Her producer thought she was not fit for TV. With this in his mind, he ended firing her on the spot. All these struggles did not deter these people from pursuing their dreams. This applies to any area in life. Be it an athlete, player, or politician, focus, and motivation affect success by a considerable amount. The question remains how can we be motivated every time? For any successful career, there are many struggles. Some call this force that offers these struggles "resistance." This resistance maintains the status quo. Everyone in life has to fight this "resistance." To be successful, we have to beat down the giant resistance. It is everywhere provided we are alive. To get over this giant, we can utilize the power of meditation.

There is a region in the brain called "thalamus." This separates consciousness from the external environment. This is the main entrance to the human consciousness. This separates the stimuli that do not need high thinking to the one that requires it. High thinking regions in the brain are cerebral cortex and subcortical areas. Our modern world has beaten our thalamus. The thalamus no longer functions properly. We are more likely to have disorders like anxiety. With this most of the time, our brains are overloaded. By utilizing the power of meditation, we can reduce the workload on our brains. Meditation assists our gate to human consciousness; it can now at least rest and rejuvenate with our mind and thalamus fully functional. This allows us to think more deeply. Since we can now think deeply, we are able to make well thought decisions and solve our issues more efficiently. Since a highly efficient brain is a focused brain. We become more focused on our daily life activities.

By meditation, we train our brains to be focused in any situation. This allows us to recover fast from failures, making everything achievable. We can use meditation to achieve our goals. The part of the brain that keeps us motivated towards our goals is known as the "dorsolateral prefrontal cortex." A study by Italian neuroscientists in 2015 found that meditation stiffens the wiliness to work towards a goal. It also builds the ability of a person to control himself/herself. This can and will, in turn, boost our motivation. The universe always expects us to produce great things. When we are more focused on our objectives, that is the ignition, and we require to start doing great things.

Chapter 4 Group Meditation

Anytime you walk upon a group of people meditating you know that you have come into the presence of a very positive energy, or something remarkable is happening.

Sometimes you can look and see hundreds of people sitting in silence with purpose, and nothing is happening except for extreme silence and deep thinking. It is very powerful to experience and witness hundreds of people practicing meditation at one time. It can be very motivating as well as doing something to your spirit that feels natural and great.

Even if you were to walk on a group of one hundred people and not know that they were meditating, not knowing exactly what they were doing, you would still be spiritually drawn to them, and you would feel that positive energy coming from the situation.

Your spirit would naturally be attracted to harmony and peace because it is very overpowering to see that much effort being put into sitting in silence without moving that is very powerful and intentional. Hundreds of people not moving with no agenda other than to be present in the powerful manifestation of positive energy in human goodness.

Meditating Sitting Down

Sitting down does not just mean being seated. It means taking your seat in a relationship with the present moment, taking your stand in your life while you are sitting. Adopting and keeping a positive posture will give you pride, which will immediately change how you look and feel about yourself. Being aware of your physical sensations and thoughts while you are sitting upright is essential to meditation while you are sitting down. Whatever emotion you may have, let it flow right through you and do not let it consume you.

We can do this anytime, in any way, just make your mind aware of it and decide you want to do it. It takes many hours of practice, and you will just want to make sure that you are comfortable and totally relaxed.

Having strength and stability can come from sitting directly on the floor and crossing your legs as you do your meditating. You can also use a large pillow or cushion, which will assist in raising your butt up off the floor to a more aligned level.

This is more about being able to concentrate and focusing on keeping your mind sitting still. Just as in meditating while lying down, establish your posture, let yourself go and allow the present moment to take charge, then awareness is immediate.

Focus on the sensations of your breath in the places of the body where they are most popular to you. Your nose and your stomach are great places to focus on to practice awareness of each breath.

Focus on the feeling of each breath as it passes through your nostrils and makes your stomach rise in and out up and down. Our minds will always wander away from our primary focus to go into something it feels is more entertaining.

This will continue to happen on a regular basis because we are human, so we can just remember to acknowledge it and remind your mind to refocus on what is important at that moment in time.

Get your mind back on the thought of your breathing and begin to expand your awareness to include sensations within the body. Whatever it is that you are feeling, be aware of that, and own it. If you feel a pain in your knee, let it be known that there is a pain in that knee, the key here is to be aware of it, so that you can move on from it.

You do not have to be consumed or held as a prisoner by it. Just sit with an awareness of those sensations, acknowledge them as pleasant or unpleasant, realizing that is exactly what you are experiencing at that moment. The breath and the body come together as a complete being at this moment, and they are seen and felt as one.

You can imagine all your thoughts and emotions like the ocean flowing peacefully and calmly. Whether you are meditating or not, it can be helpful to look at this as an excuse to sit by and take in the beautiful sounds of the ocean as we stare at the wonderfully inspiring beach.

All of the time, we are present in each moment and make sure to welcome the presence of awareness to be infinite like the birds that fly in the sky. As stated before, it will take much dedication and practice to master this, but you will benefit along the way from all of your work.

Meditating While Standing

You can meditate while standing up the same way that you are able to meditate while sitting, lying down, or walking. It is one of the four popular ways in which people all over the world are now practicing their meditation.

When you think of standing meditation, it can be helpful for you to think about a tree. I know that sounds kind of silly, but the logic is that a tree has all of the knowledge and discipline that it needs to be able to stand in one place for a very long time.

Yet trees have managed to remain in a very timeless state and are still present and in the moment with us, no matter what their age seems to be. It may help your understanding of this if you go and stand next to your favorite type of tree for a while.

Try to listen and imagine hearing exactly what the tree would be hearing at that moment. You are to try to become an immediate family with the tree so that you can understand the language in which it is communicating with the universe.

You can physically experience what the tree feels by standing barefoot on the ground and becoming one with the soil. As you share the energy of tree, soil, and universe, you will begin to feel a very natural and free type of feeling in your spirit.

The same way that it is with other types of meditation, it can help if you keep up the practice for a longer period of time than you really feel like doing it. When you get that very first impulse to quit, that is when you want to focus, dig deep and keep going.

That will serve as a very vital test of your commitment, self-control, and determination. It is not easy to accomplish at first, but you will be able to do it if you just push yourself beyond each comfort zone that you try and hold onto.

Stay consistent and do not stop trying, when you can imagine yourself being completely inside of your own body, without feeling the ground touching your feet, and the sensation of your head being elevated with a sense of grace and ease looking into the direction of the Most High who is watching us all from the heavens.

Being consciously embedded in the current state of your own life and realizing that it is vital and important that you assume and retain control of your life and the direction in which it is going.

How you stand, the way that you should hold your hands, and the posture in which you need to hold your arms are all essential to this practice. Your arms should definitely be relaxed while hanging directly along each side of your body. This stance should be held for a few moments as the awareness is claimed and stood in.

You want to be sure that you align yourself and be as centered as possible because you are going to stand strong, tall, and with much dignity. Now you have the ability to surrender yourself into just simply being with what is.

Anyone can practice standing meditation anywhere, at any time, whenever they may feel like they are ready to give it a try. Some people have tried meditation, found it too difficult or boring, or just did not understand the point of it all.

We would like to welcome back those who are willing to give it another try and who are looking to make a positive change in their lives. This can be practiced literally anytime you think about doing it. It can be while you are waiting on the elevators, while you are driving, while you are waiting on the bus or train, it is all in your mind.

Meditating While Walking

With walking, we have experienced our bodies a little bit differently than when we are sitting or lying down during meditation. Bringing our attention to our feet and using that contact between each of our feet and the ground, we can imagine it as if we are giving kisses to the world each time we step down.

When the mind wanders off while we are walking and meditating, it is no different than it is with any other meditation practice. As long as we to take note of where it went and get it back into the moment, we can continue the harmony with our breathing and our steps. Take slow strides when you are walking, and you will notice more about nature and things around you.

Walking meditation can be done at many different speeds because, the same way life can throw us into another direction, our minds will assist us with the transition from mindful walking into mindful running, and that can be very a helpful tool in the practice of meditation.

You can begin by standing still, bringing awareness to your body as a whole and realize those impulses in the mind that are going to initiate the process of walking by lifting one foot, so we become aware of each time we actually lift each foot.

Now you will get the actual impulse to finally take that first step forward, which will now begin to bring us into touch with the full aspect of each sensation that we experience in our bodies that are connected with walking, lifting the heel of the foot and the actual swinging of your leg as it is being moved forward.

Coordinating all this with our breathing while being able to observe each breath as our body moves is essential to mastering this practice. While being mindful, a useful way to coordinate this is that you can breathe in as the back of your heel raises up off of the ground and breathe out each time it touches down.

Now I want you to think of what you are going to be doing with your hands during this time. You just need to be aware of the fact that they are hanging down on the side of your body and let them rest right where they are.

There is never just one specific way to accomplish these practices. You can experiment with what feels right for you and the way that you live. There is no right or wrong way; it is all about practicing, being consistent, and finding what is comfortable for you while you are walking.

Meditating While Standing

The most challenging thing to do when you are trying to practice lying down while you meditate is staying awake. This takes more work than the actual meditation, because as soon as you get relaxed, you begin to get sleepy. You have to remember not to fall asleep because you can get so relaxed that you can fall right into drowsiness, unawareness and be out for the count before you realize it.

And without practice this happens quite a bit, most people have talked about how hard it is to actually stay awake during this process, and without practice you are going to fall into drowsiness, get sleepier and the deeper the sense of relaxation, you are asleep.

Meditating while lying down, has different types of benefits. During the early stages of meditation practice, it can definitely be more comfortable for some people. As you concentrate on your breathing, it gets easier to fill the gravity. You can, at times, feel as if you are floating, and that can bring about an extreme amount of peace.

Practicing mindfulness while you lay on your back is called Yoga by many people.

Place a padded surface like a rug, a large cushion, or even a mattress that you may have on the floor.

You can simply dedicate your focus to being on hearing, bringing back your attention to hearing over and over again when it wanders off. Just bring it back. It's a powerful way to practice coming to your senses through the sense of hearing.

Some people find it very relaxing to meditate with their eyes closed while they lay down and have stated that it is helpful in retaining awareness and easier to become focused and concentrate.

It can be very valuable if you can practice meditating while you are lying down before you fall asleep, and again as soon as you wake up. This can affect how you choose to go about your day and will determine the true intention before you even get out of bed.

You can decide that you are going to have a great day, and you will not get caught in the negativity of any circumstance or situation. That is a positive practice that you can do daily to help ensure that you have a good day.

You can do the same thing when you lay in bed at the end of the night before you go to sleep. Experience your body and your mind. Think about what happened during the craziness of your day and be aware of each of the senses you have. Plan out how you intend to relax and be at peace during your sleep, enjoy and remember your dreams.

Anytime you are laying down is a chance to work at getting stronger at this. There are constantly new possibilities for learning and growing and healing. And without realizing it once again, there are opportunities many times throughout the day that we can take a few moments to lay down and practice our mindfulness and meditation techniques.

Our bodies are in need of rehabilitation and need to learn how to live again. Sometimes this can be after we suffer an injury or an illness, and our body just needs some positive, healthy attention because it has been neglected. You can take the time to get it back to where it needs to be, paying close attention and feeling your body movement by movement sense by sense as you go through your day.

That goes back to what we said earlier about paying close attention to your body, and it will tell you exactly what it needs, and you will be able to act accordingly. We never know to the degree in which our bodies are responding to us, but it definitely will respond.

The body actually loves the process of getting all of this new attention, care, compassion, and love. It receives all of that and will return it to you with the same amount of love.

53

Chapter 5 How Does Sleep Meditation Help With Sleep?

So why does this help with sleep? What are you getting from it? Well, meditation can play a huge part in sleep, and you need sleep in order to function in life. Let's look at what sleep does for you, what meditation does for the body, and how the two of them work together.

Sleep and why we need it

Sleep is essential for daily functions in our life. If you don't have enough sleep, you're going to feel it the next day, especially in terms of production and the like.

For many people, a lack of sleep leads to less energy, and that means you're not producing as much as you could do. Sleep allows us to get the job done the next day, but it also allows us as well to mentally be there as well.

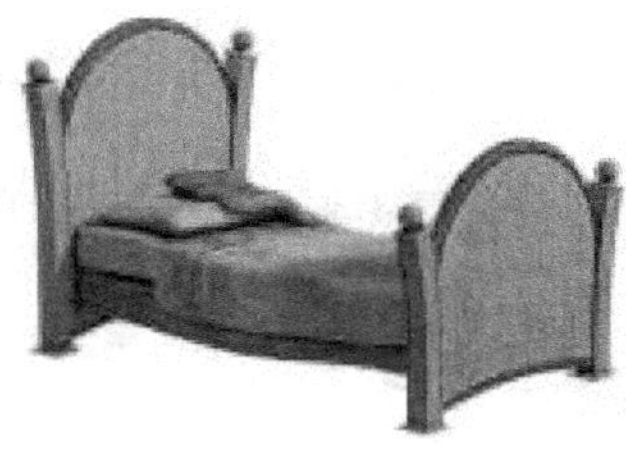

When we don't get enough sleep, we're not as sharp, and our performance suffers during the day. It can actually make things a whole lot worse for you as well. It keeps you in the present and happier in life as well.

Sleep also affects our brain waves as well. Typically, if you're anxious, you have a lot of beta brain waves, which are what are present when we need to make decisions, be attentive, or when we're anxious and uneasy, and when we have depression as well.

The negative thoughts actually can start to come forward even in the late hours of the night, and that will then make it harder for you to sleep each day, and it will cause you to have more trouble the closer you get to waking up. It's important that we get sleep, because it will help curb these problems, and make it easier for you.

Not only that, lack of sleep can cause bodily functions to start to worsen as well. our bodies will slow down, which slows our metabolic functions, and that in turn will actually cause us to gain weight, make the body work harder to do various tasks, and overall, it's just not good for you to deal with. You're going to get slower, and that can cause you to falter. It can even lead to you getting sick, the body shutting down, and if you don't sleep period for long periods of time, it can even end in death.

So yes, you need sleep in order to function as a human and have a much easier time with various tasks. It's super important, and meditation can actually help with this.

Meditation and how it helps

So how does meditation help with this. well, if you meditate, you're producing more alpha, delta, and theta brainwaves. These waves help to relax and help promote deep sleep, and you will produce less beta brainwaves as a result of this.

These brainwaves also will help us stay more refreshed in the morning as well, bringing us to the peak state we can be.

It also brings us to the present, instead of worrying about tomorrow. Do you have nights where you're always worrying? It's definitely annoying, but if you start to focus on the present when you're meditating, especially sleep meditation, you'll be able to tap into the thoughts of the fact that the day is over, right now you're sleeping, and you won't have to worry about anything but the here and now.

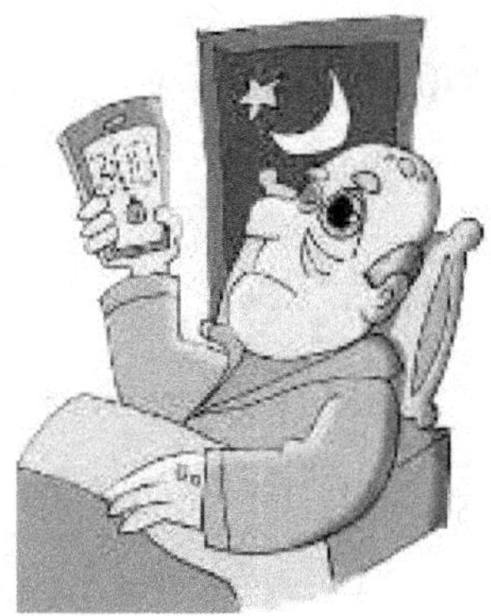

Meditation allows you to manage your brain and move it from worry to one of both comfort and of peace, which will allow you to have a relaxed mind as you begin to sleep.

With this, you're focusing the attention to the present state, and from there, you'll bring your mind into a better state of awareness regarding the emotions, thoughts, and also the physical state of this. You'll be able to manage your thoughts better, and run them way better instead of trying to let them control you.

If you do this before you go to bed, or using deep sleep meditation, you'll realize that you feel better, and you'll get a more restful, better sleep.

It also will boost melatonin as well, which is a hormone that will help regulate sleep in the body. If you do this, you'll increase this, and doing it right before bed makes it even more worthwhile. Sleep meditation does this as well, and it stimulates the pineal gland. By doing this, you'll feel way better and have a much deeper, more restful sleep.

This can be used to help supplant the use of supplements too, which might not work as quickly as good old meditation.

How Sleep Meditation helps Sleep

Meditation does wonders for the quality of sleep, particularly in the stage of REM sleep. This is definitely a huge part of improving your sleep pattern. The quality of your sleep is more important than how long you stay in bed.

If you're always tired despite putting in eight hours of sleep each day, you're not necessarily getting enough in terms of time, you actually need to have more REM stage sleep. The REM stage is actually shown by the state of the brain waves that are happening. The activity during this is similar to how you act when you're wakeful, which is the mixture between alpha and the theta waves, and the beta waves are actually more high-level thinking and concentration. This is the dream stage.

REM is the final stage of sleep, and not reaching this actually is why you feel fatigued and groggy. If you're woken up during REM sleep, you'll feel groggy as well.

The REM stage begins with the signals from the base of the brain which is called pons. Meditation actually elevates the Pons area of the brain. From this, it can be concluded that if you do meditate, you'll have a much better REM cycle and more chances to rewire and connect parts of the brain when you sleep as well. This also does explain the increase of drams as well when you begin meditation.

Meditation, allows for more imagery as well, which is what also stimulates this part of the body, making it easier for you to have a chance to experience the REM stage of dreams. Simply put, you're going to have a much better experience actually taking the time to experience REM sleep and have more restful sleep if you do meditate.

Sleep meditations allow for this to happen right away. Meditation helps to relax the body, allowing you as well to be in better control over your thoughts too. You'll have a better idea of what types of thoughts you want to have, and you can regulate these so that you're not at the mercy of them. This as well will allow you to have a much easier time with falling asleep, allowing you to feel better, and be more restful.

Sleep is so important, but in our society, it's often lost due to the fact that we all lead stressful lives. But, with meditation, you'll be able to improve the state of your life, and you'll be able to feel better, but also have a better sleep pattern as a result of what you do.

Chapter 6 Stress And Sleep Meditation

Stress is a huge factor in whether or not you're going to get restful sleep, and it actually is probably the most major culprit when it comes to insomnia. This shouldn't be that surprising, but we'll go over why that is, and how sleep meditation will allow you to relax the body, and reduce the instance of stress.

What is Stress

So, what in the world is stress? Stress is actually the "fight or flight" response when you're confronted with danger. Let's say that you're worried about an upcoming exam, or a work presentation. Maybe you start to feel a little bit apprehensive about this sort of thing, and you begin to worry a little bit. When you finally get it done, the stress tends to reduce, allowing you to feel better

But, we're often super busy and hit from all fronts with this feeling, this need to either fight or flight, and this will make us feel anxious all the time. This stress starts to compound over time, and it certainly makes it harder for you to calm down.

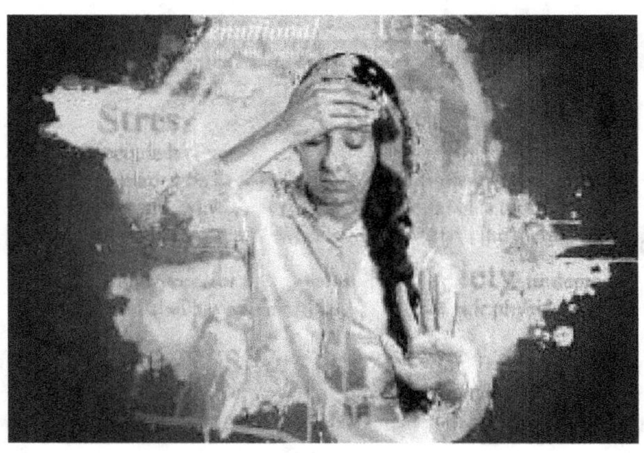

Stress releases cortisol, which elevates the heart rate, makes the beta brain waves much more prevalent, and it makes your energy levels increase. It also releases adrenaline, which is a hormone that causes your energy to increase as well, but if you start to release this all the time, it actually can start to make you feel sleepy as well, and often, messed up adrenals are a huge part of a person's problems, and stress can cause a lot of issues with this.

So yes, stress isn't good for you if you're going to be stressed all the time. Now, if you're stressed once in a while and you use that stress to propel yourself forward isn't that bad, but if you're overworking the body in this front, it can cause a lot of problems for you in the future.

Stress and Insomnia

So how does stress cause insomnia? Well, stress is something that causes cortisol to be released. Again, it will elevate the heartrate, and it's the body's response to stress. This might be good if you need a little bit of an extra push, but when you're stressed all the time, this is how the body ends up staying up late, tossing and turning and not sleeping. Your body won't be relaxed, but instead on the edge all the time.

When you sleep, instead of thinking about the present, you're worried about the future. You're worried about how that presentation is going to go, your family, your partner, your life. You might end up feeling your brain go from one element to another, almost like it's jumping from one place to another. It's not good for you, and this then causes more stress, so more cortisol will be released, and more anxiety will start to form.

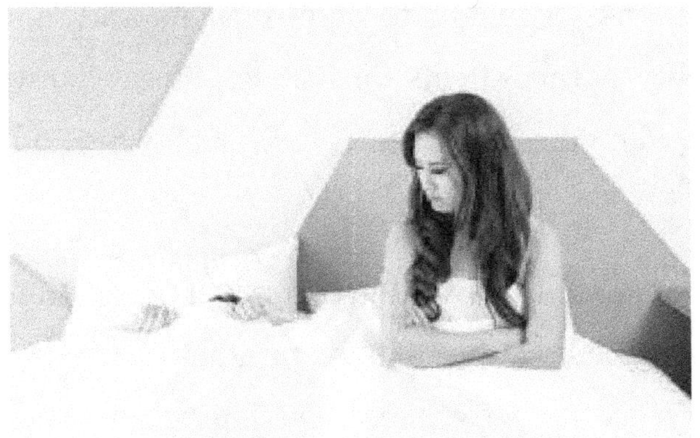

This is how insomnia is formed, and your brain just won't shut down. The best way to have a restful life, is to have restful sleep and to help curb the stress. It's important, since it actually can determine whether you're going to be going throughout the day dragging, or if you're going to be happy and restful.

If you want to sleep better, you need to curb the stress. Now, it's nearly impossible to just make stress get up and walk away. Stress will be there, but there are ways to relax the body, and meditation is actually one of the best ways to help relax it, allowing for you to feel better and to have a much better, happier life. You don't have to go through life constantly feeling stressed, especially when you're trying to sleep, so you should tap into what is making you stressed, and start to work on relaxing the body so that you're not feeling this way all the time.

Meditation helps

Meditation can do a whole lot of good on the stress in the body. It's actually a major means to help mitigate and in some cases, help to reverse the effects of stress. Stress is what causes insomnia, and meditation does a whole lot for the body in helpful ways.

How does it? Well, have you ever heard of the relaxation response? This is how the body responds to various factors that are used to relax the body, such as sedatives and the like. This is the complete opposite of the stress response, and if you're trying to help reduce the instances of stress when you're trying to sleep, it's a major part of it.

Now, the relaxation response is actually don't by you. It's a voluntary response and your ability to help your body release the chemicals. You can have this become involuntary, but it's not that easy. However, if you do this, you'll start to relegalize everything is slowing down. That's essentially what you want to do. You want to slow everything down.

This actually will cause the blood flow to move to the brain, which in turn will allow you to improve the responses that the brain makes to different factors in the body. You know what else actually does this? Drugs. Sedatives that you take before you go in for a treatment or an operation do the same thing to the body that this relaxation does.

However, with those, you get side effects, and there are a few dangers to them, which is why I don't suggest fixing your sleep responses with drugs. However, meditation helps to naturally relax the body, and it also allows you to consciously do this. That's right, you're aware this entire time, and that makes a huge difference. You're the one who's deciding to do this, and it definitely can help you improve your sleep schedule, and turn off the stress.

Guided meditations do a lot of good for a person, and guided sleep meditations will allow you to turn this on, and turn the stressors off. Usually, with these you can feel the powerful effects that these have on your sleep, and it will gently lull you into a slumbering state. You'll notice with these that they have a little bit of vocals and music that allow you to relax and fall asleep. The tracks actually help turn the brainwaves that cause you to feel stressed and anxious. Instead, you'll feel restful, and one of the best parts of it, is you don't have to deal with this for a long period of time.

For just about 10 minutes or so, these guided meditations will help lull you to sleep in the way that you want it to. With this, you'll end up being able to turn the brain off in the ways that you don't want to think, and in turn, you'll feel happier, and much better as well.

Stress is something that we can't get away from. You often can't do that sort of thing, simply because it is hard to escape. Life isn't easy, and stress is a natural response, but if you're able to use sleep meditation in order to fix this, you'll realize that not only will you feel better, but you'll be less stressed, and much happier than you've been before.

Chapter 7 Intention Setting

You need to minimize all distractions around you. To do this, you can put your phone on silent or even turn it off and let others know that you need some silence and privacy for a while.

Find a comfortable spot for yourself and sit on a comfortable chair with your feet planted firmly on the floor.

Start breathing in slowly and deeply through your nose. Inhale through your nose and exhale through your mouth.

When you feel calm and centered, bring awareness into those aspects of your life that you want to transform.

Imagine the highest vision that you have for a particular aspect of your life as if it has already happened and you are currently living in this energy. For instance, how do you look? How do you feel? What are you doing? Is there someone else with you? What is happening all around you? What are the different daily practices that you need to undertake to let your ideal vision exist?

You need to make this vision as compelling and as real as you possibly can. Your vision is not something that you need to create—it exists. You merely need to access it.

Now that you have spent some time concentrating on your breathing, the next question that you need to answer is "what is my goal?" You can have one or multiple goals. Remember that you need to concentrate on only one goal at a time. Make a mental note of all the things that you need to do to achieve your goal.

Think, "What do I need to do daily to achieve this goal?"

Think about your answer and make a mental note of it.

Make sure that your daily activities contribute to your goal.

Now that you have all the information that you need to understand your goal, the next step is to energize these steps.

Set a trajectory towards the goal you desire. Visualize yourself as you slowly sprint towards your goal.

I feel empowered, confident, and certain that I can achieve my goal.

I have the momentum to keep going towards my goal.

I will not stop until I reach my goal.

I will contribute towards my goal on a daily basis.

I have the motivation to achieve what I desire.

I am excited to work on my goal.

Visualize how wonderful it feels to achieve your goal. The feeling of calm, relaxation, and peace.

I feel calm and content.

I am happy and satisfied.

I feel confident.

I am grateful for all that I have in life.

I will continue to work on improving myself.

Now, you need to float back to reality. Spend a couple of moments and concentrate on your breathing. Hold onto the wonderful feelings you experienced a moment ago and don't let them go.

Breathe in slowly through your nose and exhale.

Breathe in and breathe out.

Breathe in and breathe out.

You will end this meditation on the count of five.

One, two, three, four, and five.

Once you are awake, make a note of all this in a journal. Try to be as detailed as you can. You can always go back to your visualization whenever you need some motivation, or you need to remind yourself of your goals. Use your visualization to focus on your goals and to ignore all unnecessary things.

Chapter 8 Meditation For Happiness

I want to welcome you to this exercise that will help you cultivate happiness and feel happy.

Find yourself something comfortable to wear.

You can either lie down or sit. You can sit in a chair or sit on the ground with your legs crossed. Let your hands rest in your lap or by your side.

If you feel uncomfortable at any time, you can immediately stop the recording. You simply need to open your eyes, and the meditation ends.

Now, close your eyes and listen to my voice.

Let your mind be free to explore, to smile, and experience happiness.

Concentrate only on your breathing and nothing else.

Your breaths start to become slower and deeper.

Breathe in through your nose and exhale through your mouth. While you breathe in and out, permit yourself to let go of the outside world.

Visualize a path in your mind's eye. The path can be anything, but at the end of the path, you need to visualize a door. This door opens up the path to your inner world.

Push the door open, and you can see bright light all around you. The light feels warm, welcoming, and it helps you relax.

Your inner world is full of bright color, and it is time for you to step into this wonderful world.

Relax into all the warmth and peace that exists within.

You are the only one that knows this place, and it is your safe haven.

Take a deep breath and shut the door.

Enter this world, immerse yourself in it, and forget all about the external world for a while. This is your personal world of peace and love. You feel safe and happy in here.

This is your time to work on your happiness. Let happiness spread within your body so that it eventually radiates from you.

It is okay even if your mind starts to wander. It is all right even if you realize that your thoughts have gone off on a tangent.

Remember that you are in charge of your thoughts and if you feel like your thoughts are wandering, then you can bring awareness back. Listen to the sound of my voice and concentrate only on my voice.

Now, take a deep breath and start to relax your body.

Start with your feet. Will your toes to relax and then your feet.

Feel your legs relax slowly. Now, feel the muscles in your thigh and then the ones in your abdomen relax.

Gently allow them to relax.

Start to focus on your chest. Focus on the muscles around your ribcage and let them relax before you move onto your back.

You can now feel the muscles in your shoulders relax. All the tension that you feel disappears.

Now, allow the muscles in your neck relax and move towards your head.

Take a deep breath and allow your entire body to relax.

Your breath fills up your lungs with oxygen.

Start to exhale slowly until there is no air in your lungs.

Breathe in through your nose for a count of four.

One, two, three, and four.

Hold your breath for a count of two.

One and two.

Exhale through your mouth for a count of eight.

One, two, three, four, five, six, seven, and eight.

Breathe in, hold your breath, and breathe out.

Imagine the path that you took to enter your inner world.

Walk on that path once again, and you are now surrounded by the same bright light that you saw.

Walk on the path that leads you through an evergreen forest. There are pine trees that line the path on either side. The morning sun is shining brightly, and it is casting golden rays of warm sunlight. Continue to walk on this path, and you will find a rock outcropping overlooking a landscape of mountains.

You are surrounded by hundreds of mountain peaks all, and some seem to be closer than the rest. Gaze at this beautiful scenery in front of you and let the feeling of peace wash all over you.

Appreciate the beauty of nature that's all around you and be thankful for it.

Enjoy the view and give yourself a moment to smile. Take in the beauty that's present before you.

The golden rays of the warm sunlight are illuminating the landscape. The colors are gently mixing with each other all around you, and it looks like a beautiful painting painted by a maestro. Smile and become aware of all that's around you.

Imagine the sounds of birds chirping around you. Enjoy the symphony of the sounds of nature all around you. Take it all in and smile.

Now, you will notice a large tree near you. The tree seems quite old, and it has a large trunk. Visualize this tree in great detail. The bark of the tree looks like that of a sweet birch, and its leaves have a sweet smell to them.

A gentle wind is blowing through the forest, and it blows a couple of leaves away from the tree. One such leaf lands in your palm and you smile as the leaf gives off a slight sweet-smelling minty scent.

Smile at the beauty of nature and take a deep breath. Breathe in all the happiness that you feel and breathe out all your worries.

Breathe in and breathe out.

The leaves start to rustle gently all around you. Light and airy sounds surround you.

Everything around you complements one another, and everything seems to be in sync. This synchronization of nature makes you happy and makes you smile.

You are now surrounded by the warm and the wonderful sounds.

Listen to the music of nature; you can feel your heart fill up with joy. You are surrounded by beauty, and it makes you feel happy.

Look around; there is a bush with bright green leaves next to the tree. The leaves resemble that of a maple tree, but the bush is filled with small berries like blackberries.

Go ahead and pick a few berries. Now you can eat these tasty-looking berries.

Enjoy the flavors of these berries and savor how wonderful they taste. Start to slowly chew and then swallow these delicious berries.

You can feel the warmth and energy radiate from your core as these berries slide down your throat and into your tummy.

You can feel energy and strength rise within you. This energy spreads from your stomach to your entire body. You can feel this brilliant energy radiating throughout your body. All your senses feel happy.

You feel a sense of relaxation and appreciation wash all over you.

Look at the nature that's present all around you. Take in the warmth of the sunlight, the chirping of the birds, the greenery, and the wonderful scents all around you. Allow yourself to soak up all this goodness and wonder.

This powerful energy continues to course through your body.

It is pure energy that makes you smile.

Bask in this wonderful energy. Let it wash over every cell in your body. Let your body be infused with nature's wonderful energy.

Stay in this place for a couple of moments and smile more.

Now that your body is infused with this wonderful energy, it is time for you to return to the reality.

Your inner world has equipped you with all that you need to feel energized and happy when you return to the outer world.

You can visit your inner world whenever you feel low or dull. You can always come back to this inner sanctum of yours and feel good about yourself.

Take a deep breath and bid goodbye to this wonderful place for now. Hold onto the energy that this place gave you. Hold onto the feelings of positivity and happiness.

You feel good about yourself, and you are looking forward to going back to your world.

As you walk, you will notice the door to the outer world. Slowly open the door, take a deep breath, and step inside.

You are now back in the real world, and you are full of happiness and positivity.

Breathe in slowly and deeply.

Take a deep breath through your nose and hold it for a count of four.

One, two, three, and four.

Now, breathe out through your mouth and hold it for the count of eight.

One, two, three, four, five, six, seven, and eight.

Take another deep breath through your nose and exhale through your mouth.

Start to slowly open your eyes and feel the energy of the inner world shine brightly in your body.

Take a deep breath, smile, and return to your day.

You can follow this exercise whenever you want a burst of happiness. It will help you appreciate all that is good in your life and let go of your worries.

Chapter 9 Meditation For Heart

Meditation that comes from the heart, and for the heart is important because it can help you lead a life full of wellness, and happiness as well. Here, you'll learn about the best meditation for the heart that is possible, and some important aspects that come from this too.

Why Meditation for Heart?

The heart is a vital part, and it allows for you to open up your mind, and body in a much better way. Your heart has a chakra that vibrates, and with the right amount of resonance, it can exude a calmness that will help you.

So, how do you meditate for the heart? What is an excellent meditation that will help with this? Good thing you're here because you're about to find out in this chapter!

A simple Meditation to Open the Heart

To help you open the heart, you begin with the following. Sit in a comfy position, close your eyes, and proceed to breathe in, and breathe out, just like how we mentioned before, and as you breathe in and breathe out, let go of all the gunk that's stuck inside of you. Picture that it's a new day, a new time period, so you don't want to carry the old stuff with you.

Take one hand and put it on the heart, and then one on the belly. As you breathe, pay mind to how comfy this feels, and be aware that you can do this whenever to help take care of yourself.

At this point, you can pay note to your breathing, and how it calms you, how it lets you go of yesterday, and how it gives you that feeling of safety. As you do this, realize you're here for yourself, and as you release the tensions of yesterday, let your attention come to this day. Pay attention to the hour, the time that you're in, and pay attention to your day, and how it's going to be incredible.

Keep your heart open, and picture letting the universe coming in.

Finally, finish off with some breathing in, and then breathing out, and slowly open your eyes.

This is a good one to first awaken the heart, and it is a great one for starting the day.

Meditating to connect with the heart's energy

This is a seven-step process to help you connect with the energy from the heart, and it's both simple, yet truly effective. To begin, you sit in a position that is comfortable, and from there, close your eyes.

Let the thoughts of the outside world go, even if for a moment.

Once they are gone, focus on the spiritual heart center, which is the middle of your chest, where the heart is. Become aware that the heart is well a space and a point of awareness where feelings come in and leave. At the base of it, the heart is empty, and there are peace and subtle light. You may picture this light, whether it be white, gold, pink, or blue. don't strain though, just take in whatever is there.

At this point, put your attention on the center of the heart, and from there breathe in a gentle manner and let the breath flow to the heart, picturing a soft, pastel light moving into the chest, where the heart is.

Next, you should let the breath go inwards, and then outwards, and from there, ask your heart what it must say. don't phrase it as an order, but instead, a general statement that you want your heart to express itself.

At this point, you'll want to sit and listen for about 5-10 minutes. Listen to your heart, and it will release various emotions, wishes, fears, and memories, and there is a lot in there. You will find yourself paying attention.

If there is a strong emotion, you might feel he breath change, but experience what it is, and if you feel yourself daydream, bring the attention back to the center of the heart.

When you're done, you should thank the heart for what it says, and let the thoughts and feelings go. The feelings that come up are often repressed, and this is a way to purify the heart. It is healthy, and when you're done, open your eyes and breathe. You'll feel refreshed, and better than ever before.

A Meditation for Opening the Heart

This is a great one to help you open yourself up and build more kindness. we'll discuss compassion and kindness in mediation in the next chapter, but before you begin, you must open your heart, and that's the generalized purpose of this mediation.

To begin, you should find a place where you can be not interrupted and give yourself time without various distractions. At this point, sit down, close your eyes, and breathe. Once you've gotten comfy, you should recall something that is challenging or difficult, whatever is causing you stress. Feel free to experience the struggle, emotional discomfort, or distress. At this point, become aware that this is a moment of discomfort and struggle, and you can acknowledge that it is stressful, haunting, painful, or you might speak the words that you feel.

You will want to recognize the struggle, stress, and what you're suffering, and realize that it's a part of life that will link you to the humanity that you have. However, don't let this overwhelm you. Remember, you're not alone, and that others have struggled in the same way that you have.

At this point, put your hands on top of the heart. Take some deep breaths, relax the tension that you're holding, and when you breathe out, feel the stress as it disperses and leaves the body, along with the warm and gentle touch from the hearts that are on the chest. Feel the comforting feeling of the light building within the hands, spreading to the heart. At this point, let this energy flow from you, spreading out.

At this moment, you should ask yourself what you need to hear and feel right now in order to provide kindness to yourself. You can ask if you can be kind to yourself, forgive, be strong, be compassionate, learn to accept yourself, be patient, and give yourself the compassion that you need.

Repeat this and continue to speak this. Feel the energy start to disperse and change, and when you're done, thank your heart as you come out of this, and you'll start to realize that your heart is open, and you'll be able to put together the self-compassion that you'll need when you need it the most. This is the best way to clear away blocks, open up the heart, and feel better.

Meditation for heart will allow you to relax and become a better person than you want to be, and it's a great way to help you improve on your own personal character and let go of the past so that you can be happier, and brighter as well.

Chapter 10 The First Steps To Ending The Insomnia Struggle

Insomnia, in medical terms, is one of the massive diseases worldwide. Insomnia statistics are growing every day. Today, about 29% of men, 37% of women, 25% of children, and 75% of pregnant women suffer from this disease. Insomnia is expressed in disturbed sleep. Patients are far from always seriously taking insomnia and simply let their treatment "go" on its own. This attitude leads to unpleasant and dangerous consequences in the form of the transition of the disease into a chronic form, neurological disorders, pathologies of internal organs, and mental disorders. Not everyone can cope with insomnia on their own, and in most cases, to get a good result, the help of a medical specialist is needed.

Insomnia, in short, is a widespread phenomenon that is a violation of the quality and quantity of sleep, adversely affecting human daily activities.

Occasionally, it happens in each of us. But when a person spends night after night without sleep - this is a completely different matter. Insomnia is almost always a reflection of other disorders. It testifies either to failures in the physical state, or to emotional experiences.

Often, chronic diseases accompanied by pain (say, arthritis) do not give an opportunity to close your eyes for a moment. After a quarrel with your soul mate, you can also spend the night without sleep. And the troubles at work can turn into the fact that a person tosses and turns under the covers until morning.

In addition, sometimes, there are enough changes in the usual rhythm of life to cause sleep disturbances. For example, due to work on the night shift or because of different time zones.

According to experts, insomnia often begins with a few nights when it is not possible to fall asleep, say, after an injury or emotional upheaval. After such nights, snacking during the day can become a habit, and at night, unsuccessful attempts to fall asleep. A person begins to watch television programs while lying in bed or to visit the refrigerator in the middle of the night. Before he has time to realize what is happening to him, new habits acquire a systematic character. Such disorders are known as habitual insomnia.

All the efforts made by most people to normalize sleep, in reality, only worsen it. The root causes disappear, and insomnia, sadly, remains. Bad habits are fixed that don't allow a person to fall asleep: people begin to constantly look at their watches; as the night closes in, they become anxious.

The sleep rhythm of people suffering from chronic insomnia is so unsettled that they resemble one frantically dancing to the measured melody of an old waltz. What are the signs of chronic insomnia?

- You have difficulty falling asleep almost every evening for several weeks.

- You are overwhelmed with fear of going to bed because you doubt whether you can fall asleep.

- You feel very tired during the day and cannot concentrate in order to work normally.

- You resort to alcohol or medication in order to fall asleep.

Positive Thinking

It is necessary to have a positive attitude not only to oneself but also to life. No doctor can give us health if we ourselves do not take an active part in the process of our own healing. Man must enjoy life. I want to teach you how to use positive thinking to defeat your illnesses.

The point of power is here and now - in our head. And it doesn't matter how long ago negative thoughts began to prevail in us, relations with others deteriorated, finances ran out, self-hatred appeared, and illness came. It's never too late to start changing. Until now, our life and our experience have been created by the thoughts that we kept in mind, as well as those words that we constantly used. Nevertheless, such thinking now belongs to the past; we have already overcome this line. What our tomorrow, the day after tomorrow, the next week, month, year, etc., depends on our current, momentary thoughts and words. The point of application of force is always in the current moment.

Now - this is when we begin to change our lives. What a liberating thought! We can begin to part with the old nonsense. Right now. Even the smallest initial step can be decisive. Here are the first steps to getting rid of insomnia, at whatever stage it might be.

Autogenic Training

The basic principles of autogenic training were developed by the German neuropathologist Johannes Heinrich Schultz at the beginning of the 19th century. Having published several articles in special journals, in 1932, he presented to the medical community, his method described in the monograph "Autogenic training - concentrated self-relaxation."

According to Schultz, auto-training is more suitable for people of an intellectual type, who also have the necessary perseverance. However, in this book, I aim to familiarize you with simple natural techniques that will be useful for improving your well-being. In this case, self-help is understood as a conscious decision to join in the simplified exercises outlined here.

A characteristic feature of autogenous training is the gradual mastery of certain exercises in order to learn how to control the work of internal organs and achieve mental and physical relaxation.

Along with other factors, two fundamental observations served as the impetus for creating an autogenic training. The first is the establishment by Oskar Vogt of the fact that a person who is able to bring himself into a hypnotic state can achieve "deep peace and complete rest" in this way. In this sense, autogenic training is also a way of switching the body from an intense working state to a state of rest. One of the goals of the exercises is to make this transition as inconspicuous and fleeting as possible - "in no time."

In the process of self-hypnosis, a change of state occurs in a strictly defined, unchanging sequence, namely:

1. The necessary posture is taken, and relaxation sets in.

2. The eyes are closed.

3. There is a feeling of general reassurance.

4. A feeling of heaviness appears.

5. There is a pleasant sensation of a feeling of warmth spreading throughout the body.

Exercises

As outlined, we shall start the following exercises:

1. Taking the right pose.

2. The closure of the eyelids.

3. Achieving a sense of comfort.

4. Development of a feeling of heaviness.

5. Nap.

It must be remembered that clothing must be comfortable, not interfering with concentrated self-relaxation. The collar must be unfastened, a tie, a belt, tight shoes to relax or remove.

Pose

For classes, you need to choose a position so that "whenever possible, eliminate any mechanical stress." The body should be completely relaxed and be in it without the use of muscular effort. For auto-training, the following three poses are recommended.

1. "Reclining": This position is best taken in a chair deep enough, with a high back, so that the lower back is located comfortably, and it would be possible to conveniently tilt your head. The armrests should be at such a height that you can put slightly bent elbows on them.

2. "Sitting": An ordinary chair of the appropriate height with a not too soft seat is suitable for this pose. The center of gravity falls on the pelvis or ischium. At the same time, the loin is straightened, and the upper body is slightly bent and resembles the bent back of a cat. The head is relaxed and lowered perpendicular to the pelvis, not the femur. Otherwise,

the stomach will be squeezed. The legs are placed at shoulder level, hands are resting on the knees without stopping, and the hands hang freely between the hips: like a coachman who relaxed, weakened the reins, and his horses rave by themselves. If the wrists are completely relaxed, then this is a sure sign that the body position is chosen correctly.

The pose is widely used in group exercises.

3. "Lying": A comfortable, free posture is taken, with the head resting on a pillow. The legs are extended; you can't cross your legs. The feet are slightly outward, which helps to relieve muscle tension. The arms are extended along the torso with palms down and slightly bent at the elbows.

Eyelid Closure

Eyes are closed only after the correct relaxed posture has been adopted. Along with other factors, the meaning of closing the eyelids is to turn off optical irritation, so that during the next exercise - achieving calm - you can use projection in the dark if necessary.

In this case, you should not make any special, deliberate movements of the eyeball, such as looking up and inside. It is only a matter of simply closing the eyes.

Reaching Calm

Only now is the time to move on to "general tuning formulas" (according to Schulz). "Configuring" is carried out using the phrase: "I am completely calm." This phrase is necessary while maintaining the relaxation of the body with eyes closed, to "create" in your imagination as distinctly as possible. It turns out that the phrase can occur in the imagination in various forms, depending on the personality characteristics of the person.

Imagination can be "optical" when a person sees this phrase as if written "in the dark space of the eye" (projection in the dark), or acoustic, in which it is perceived in the form of sound, often with different and variable stresses. If the graphic or sound form has a distinct rhythm, then the person, at least partially, belongs to the artistic type. Representatives of a purely artistic type can recreate this phrase in the form of an image, rhythm, pulsation, etc. And finally, there is a sharply expressed mental type of people, "whose form of imagination does not rely upon or is only limited to rely on sensually-shaped phenomena."

Schulz strongly emphasizes that the phrase mentioned is solely intended to bring into a state of drowsiness and in no case, should be taken as a "calming exercise."

The development of a feeling of heaviness

As already mentioned, the phrase "I am completely calm" is not an exercise for training. It serves only to tune your own "I."

The center of consciousness is intended for thought, which is currently being inspired. If the exercise is successful, then in the corresponding arm, lying calmly, a sensation of muscle heaviness really appears. But an attempt (out of curiosity or for control) to raise this hand leads to the exact opposite effect - the hand seems quite light. The feeling of heaviness arises in this case due to relaxation.

When the exercise is successful, the muscles are completely relaxed and supple.

Exit from the Nap State

The first lesson in an autogenic training course ends with the development of a sensation of muscle heaviness. If, after finishing this exercise, you try to get up immediately, this can lead to various unpleasant consequences. Therefore, it is very important to correctly get out of the state. It must be remembered that you are actually in a state of self-hypnosis, although your consciousness is not turned off. The physical part of your "I" is also in a more or less deep hypnotic state, like a hypnotized body.

The exit from autogenic immersion is carried out in three stages:

1. It is necessary several times to bend sharply and unbend the arm, heavy as a result of self-hypnosis.

2. Take a deep, full breath.

3. And only then open your eyes.

The sequence of action when exiting a nap must be observed very accurately and strictly. In no case should you treat it carelessly? It is an integral part of the auto-training process and is as important as the previous steps. With this sequence, a person returns to a normal awake state.

After the correct exit from a nap, the first lesson ends. In exactly two weeks, according to Schultz, one can achieve a "satisfactory generalization" of good feelings. Only after this can we move on to the next step - developing a sensation of a feeling of warmth.

Chapter 11 Positive Affirmations For Better Sleep

An affirmation is an affirming statement that you make to yourself in order to reiterate the importance of an idea. Throughout the day, you might think of negative affirmations that validate your perspective. These can include things like, "I'm not good enough," or "Nothing is going right in my life." These statements aren't necessarily the whole truth, but they might have a certain element that can help solidify one perspective.

These affirmations are going to help you focus on what's most important and remember the ideas needed in order to get your best night's sleep possible. Repeat these back to yourself, write them down and make notes around your home, or simply remember them in your mind when you need them the most.

Affirmations For Falling And Staying Asleep

The best way to include these affirmations in your life is to repeat them daily. They will help retrain your brain to think more positively rather than the negative ways that you might be thinking now.

In order to reiterate the importance of affirmations, including physical activity can help you to remember them even more. When you integrate a physical exercise with a mental thought, it helps make it more real. It will be easier to accept these affirmations in your life when an emphasis is put on truly believing them.

The first movement that you can do in order to remember these exercises is to physically hold an item. It can be something as small as a stone that you keep in your pocket, or you can pick out a special pillow or blanket that you choose to use with each affirmation that we list throughout the following sections.

As you are saying these affirmations, physically touch and hold these items. Let it remind you of reality. Stay focused and grounded on remembering the most important aspects of these affirmations.

Alternatively, try implementing new breathing exercises that we haven't tried yet. The method of breathing in through your nose and out through your mouth is important, but as we go further, there are other ways that you can include healthy breathing with these positive sleep affirmations.

One method is by breathing through alternate nostrils. Make a fist with your right hand with your thumb and pinky sticking out. Take your pinky and place it on your left nostril, closing it so that you can only breathe through one.

Now, breathing for five counts through that nostril.

Then, take your right thumb, and place it on your right nostril, closing that and releasing your pinky from the other nostril. Now, breathe out for five.

You will notice that doing this breathing exercise on its own is enough to help you be more relaxed. Now, when you pair it with the affirmation that we're about to read aloud, you will start to put more of an emphasis on creating thinking patterns around these affirmations.

An alternate method of breathing is to breathe in for three counts, say the affirmation, and then breathe out for three counts. You can do this on your own with the affirmations that are most important to your life.

It will be beneficial for you to have a journal that you keep affirmations in as well. Have one handy to write these affirmations down as they apply to your life. Writing about them will help you remember them and keep a note of the things that are most effective in your life.

When you are having a bad day, you can visit these affirmations. When you need a little confidence booster, or some motivation, use these affirmations.

We will now get into the reading of these. Remember to focus on your breathing as we take you through these, and if you are not planning on drifting off to sleep once they have finished, taking notes can help as well.

Healthy Sleep Dedication

1. I am dedicated to making healthy choices for my sleeping habits.

2. The things that I do throughout my day will affect how I sleep; therefore, I am going to make sure to focus on making the best choices for all aspects of my health.

3. I will do things that aren't always easy because it will be in the best interest of my health overall.

4. When I am well-rested, everything else in my life become easier.

5. I am more focused when I have slept an entire night, so I know that falling asleep is incredibly important to my health.

6. Developing healthy habits is easy when I dedicate my time towards a better future.

7. It feels good to take care of myself.

8. I deserve a good night's sleep; therefore, I deserve everything else that will come along with this benefit.

9. I am naturally supposed to get rest. It is not wrong for me to be tired and to choose to do healthy things for my sleep cycles.

10. Dreams are normal, and I am focused on embracing them and avoiding nightmares.

11. I choose to go to bed at a decent time at night because it is best for my health.

12.   Whatever is waiting for me tomorrow will still be there whether I get a full night's sleep or not, so it is best to ensure I am getting the proper amount of rest.

13.   I take care of my body because I know that it is the only one that I will ever have.

14.   I allow discipline in my life to guide me in the right direction to make the choices that are healthiest for my individual and specific lifestyle.

15.   I nourish my body and make sure I get the right amount of nutrients to keep me energized throughout the day.

16.   I am strong because I get the right amount of sleep.

17.   Getting the right kind of sleep is good for my mental health.

18.   I am happier when I am well-rested. I am in a better mood and can laugh more easily when I have had a good night's sleep.

19.   I am grateful for my opportunity to be healthier and to get better sleep.

20.   I am thankful that I have the ability to make the right choices for my health and overall well-being.

21.   Having habits is not a bad thing, I just need to make sure that my habits are healthy ones.

22.   I am less stressed out when I am able to get a better night's sleep.

23.   I am the best version of myself when I am healthy. I am healthiest when I am well-rested and focused on getting a better night's sleep.

24.   Everything else in my life will fall into place as I focus on getting the best night's sleep possible.

25.   I love myself, therefore I am going to put an emphasis on dedication to better sleeping habits so that I can feel better all the time.

Relaxing

1. I am feeling relaxed.

1. Relaxation is a feeling I can elicit, not a state that I have to be in depending on certain restrictions.

2. I can feel the relaxation in my mind first and foremost.

3. As I feel my body becoming relaxed, I can feel that serenity pass through the upper half of my body.

4. All of the tension that I might have built throughout the day is now starting to fade away.

5. I am focused on myself and centered within my body.

6. I can tell that my muscles are becoming more and more relaxed.

7. There is nothing that is concerning me at the moment.

8. There will always be stressors in my life, but right now, I do not have to worry about any of those.

9. As I focus on being calmer, it is easier for my mind to relax.

10. I do not have to be afraid of what happened in the past.

11. I cannot change the things that are already written in history.

12. I don't need to be fearful of the future.

13. I can make assumptions, but my predictions will not always be accurate.

14. I can focus on the now, which is the most important thing to do.

15. As I start to draw my attention to the present moment, I find it easier to relax.

16. The more relaxed I am, the easier it will be for me to fall asleep.

17. The faster I fall asleep, the more rest that I can get.

18. I have no concern over what is going on around me. The only thing I am concerned with is being relaxed in the present moment.

19.   I exude relaxation and peace. Others will notice how quiet, calm, and collected I can be.

20.   I am balanced in my stress and pleasure aspects, meaning that I have less anxiety.

21.   I am not afraid of being stressed.

22.   Stress helps me remember what is most important in my life.

23.   Stress keeps me focused on my goals.

24.   I do not let this stress consume me.

25.   I manage my stress in healthy and productive ways.

26.   I have the main control over the stress that I feel. No one else is in charge of my feelings.

27.   It is normal for me to be peaceful.

28.   I allow this lifestyle to take over every aspect, making it easier to have a more relaxed sleep.

29.   When I can truly calm myself down all the way, it will be easier to stay asleep.

30.   I let go of my anxiety because it serves me no purpose.

31.   I am excited for the future.

32.   I am not afraid of any of the challenges that I might face.

33.   It is easy for me to be more and more relaxed.

34.   There is nothing more freeing than realizing that I do not have to be anxious over certain aspects in my life.

35.   I will sleep easier and more peacefully knowing that there is nothing in this world that I need to be afraid of.

Staying Asleep

1. Nothing feels better than crawling into my bed after a long day.

2. My bedroom is filled with peace and serenity. I have no trouble drifting off to sleep.

3. Everything in my room helps me to be more relaxed.

4. I feel safe and at peace knowing that I am protected in my room.

5. I have no trouble falling asleep once I am able to close my eyes and focus on my breathing.

6. I make sure all of my anxieties are gone so that I can fall asleep easier.

7. When bad thoughts come into my head, I know how to push them away so that I can focus instead on getting a better night's sleep.

8. I am centered on reality, which involves getting the best sleep possible.

9. It is so refreshing to wake up after a night of rest that was uninterrupted.

10.   Any time that I might wake up, I have no trouble knowing how to get myself back to sleep.

11.   Whenever I wake up, it is easy to get out of bed within the first few times that my alarm clock rings.

12.   The better night's sleep I get, the easier it is for me to wake up.

13.   I release all of the times that I have had a restless night's sleep.

14.   No matter how many times I have struggled with my sleep in the past, I know that I am capable of getting the best night's sleep possible.

15.   My sleep history doesn't matter now. I want to get a good night's sleep, so I will.

16.   The more I focus on falling and staying asleep, the fresher I will feel in the morning.

17.   Getting a good night's sleep helps me look better as well. My hair is bouncier, my face is fresher, my eyes are wider, and my smile is bigger.

18.   Sleep is something that I need.

19.   Sleep is something that I deserve.

20.   No matter how little work I got done in a day, or how much more I might have to do the next day, I need to get sleep.

21.	There is no point in my life where sleep would be entirely bad for me. It's like drinking water. I could always at least use a little bit of it.

22.	I am alert when I am focused on sleeping better.

23.	It is easier to remember the important things I need to keep stored in my memory when I have been able to have a full night's sleep.

24.	I can focus on what is going on around me more when I have been able to sleep through the night.

25.	There is nothing about getting sleep that is bad for me. As long as I am doing it in a healthy way, it will improve my life.

26.	I know how to cut out bad sleeping habits.

27.	I understand what is important to start doing to get a better sleep.

28.	As soon as I start to lay down, I am focused on drifting away.

29.	I do not let anxious thoughts keep me awake anymore.

30.	I will sleep healthy from here on out because I know that it is one of the most important decisions for my health that I can make.

Chapter 12 Deep Sleep Hypnosis

Welcome.

This is going to be a thirty-minute guided hypnosis session to help you drift off into a deep and relaxing sleep. The most important thing to do while listening to this session is to keep an open mind. You must go with the flow, listen to my voice, and remember to breathe. Remember, it is not always possible to enter a light hypnotic state on the first try, but we are going to try as I guide you gently and smoothly into this state so you can fall asleep. Please bear in mind that you are not going to enter any sort of deep catatonic state. Nothing is going to be physically altered within the realm of your mind. The process of hypnosis and this guided meditation is extremely safe, and you are in control of it.

Now, I want you to get comfortable. Because you are trying to achieve a deep sleep, you should be lying down, your head resting on your most comfortable pillow and you are warmed by your softest blanket. Lie back and let your shoulders go slack, relaxing against the cushion of your bed. Gently close your eyes and release all the tension from your muscles. Release the tension in your arms, then your legs. Let go of the tension in your chest and in your back. All of the muscles in your body begin to feel looser and looser and your body is feeling light.

Recognize that this is a time for only you. You have set aside all of your day's activities and are now ready to fully embrace a beautiful and peaceful sleep. Breathe in this moment of relaxation, where nothing else matters. There is only you in the warmth of your bed.

As you lay, I will ask you something very simple. In your mind's eye, imagination a kind of ruler or some sort of measuring device. Imagine something which can measure the depth of your own relaxation. Imagine this ruler in the front of your mind. Perhaps it is your favorite color, smooth with small painted tick marks and numbers.

Take a moment to notice where you are on your current level of relaxation. Out of a scale of 100 down to 0 being your most relaxed state. Understand that there is no right or wrong measurement to begin with. Explore your state, be honest with yourself as you measure your relaxation. What tensions do you still have left in your body? What anxieties, sadness, or pain still lingers? Very soon you are going to increase your relaxation and melt away this negativity and drift off into a peaceful sleep.

Perhaps are currently at a 60 on your scale of relaxation. Even though you may actually be lower down than that, imagine yourself moving the marker in front of you. With each deep breath, you slide the marker further down along this ruler closer and closer towards zero, towards immense relaxation. As you breathe and the marker slides down, you feel your muscles release in your arms then your legs, your back relaxes, and your chest opens like a flower, welcoming in big and tranquil breaths.

You may be aware that your sense of relaxation has expanded inside of you. Perhaps all the way down to 40 or 30. You see the marker slowly glide downwards along the scale. You feel that a wave of warmth has washed over you and you are beginning to feel your whole body becoming engulfed in the warmth of peace. As you feel your body releasing its tension even more now, you feel calmer. You have now reached a ten on your scale and gently, you take a deep breath through your nose. Let it fill your stomach until it is like to burst. Then release it.

You reach nine...You enter a peaceful, calm environment.

You reach eight...You can feel the warmth of the sun on your face. It is a reminder that you are loved.

You reach seven...Each sound that you hear, you do not deny. Instead it lulls you further and deeper into a deep state of relaxation.

You reach six...You inhale through your nose and fill your belly. You inhale all of the good things the world has to offer.

You reach five...Gently, through your nose, you release your breath. You expel any negative feelings that remain.

You reach four...You feel your body becoming lighter. Your arms and legs feel weightless and free.

You reach three...You feel your chest brimming with warmth and light.

You reach two... You accept the peace that has enveloped you. This peace welcomes you into a deepening serenity as your mind quiets.

You reach one... You feel yourself drawn towards the warmth of peaceful sleep, so close you can almost graze it with your fingertips.

You reach zero... You feel a comfort deep within you that starts in your chest and radiates outwards like a blooming flower. This comfort fills you with security and you remember that you are safe. You have released your worries and concerns, and in its place, there is warmth, light, and comfort.

Gently you are lulled by this wave of serenity. You feel yourself beginning to drift beyond zero, into a realm of warm colors. Billows of reds and pinks, yellows and oranges undulate around you in soft embraces until you float down onto a plush, cool surface.

With only your fingertips, you detect that you have landed on a grassy field. Around you, you can smell the sweet fragrance of wildflowers that have populated this clearing. Your body and mind have quieted to listen to the soft rustle of the breeze through grass and flower petals, and you remember the beauty of the earth. You breathe in through your nose a deep breath that fills your stomach. Through your nose, you slowly release it.

You recognize the warm colors from before, now painted in the sky. The reds fade into pinks seamlessly as though crafted by a painter's brush. The hues swirl into the setting sun and exude a warmth that you feel throughout your body. You are existing in this space with only beauty. You are existing without concern for time or worry. There is only you in this space and all of the tranquility it shares with you.

The pinks give way to magentas, then onto violets and dark blues. The sun sets and reveals an endless sky, sprinkled with thousands of twinkling stars. You see dustings of silver and purple in the sky. The bright sliver of moon casts its beam upon you, cascading you in comfort.

Your muscles seem to melt, going slack and welcoming sleep. The stars above you dance, twirling through the vast stretch of sky, but you are still. You allow this positive energy to enter your mind. It swells within you until you feel peace exuding from every pore. You have reached a depth of serenity that exists on the brink of sleep. Allow yourself to accept rest.

Underneath the moon, you accept rest. Soon, you begin to notice a new pleasing sensation that arrives at your arms and spreads to your legs and your back, your neck, and forehead. You recognize this sensation as a sublime floating energy entering your body. You feel a delicate tingle throughout your body, ushering in lightness and calmness. This sensation is like a soft white linen, cleansing you from the inside out. It is a warm touch of healing energy, of love and passion.

These soft vibrations rid you of tension. Anxieties are expelled. Sadness and fear no longer exist here. All of the leftover stress is now dissolving entirely, turning into dust carried off by the wind. It is melting away under the power of this healing energy. In its place there is safety and the knowledge that you are loved by whom you love. It is merely you, the stars, and the moon.

The lightness you feel swells, as if tiny balloons are attached to different parts of your body. You feel your body beginning to rise and drift upwards in the direction of the stars. Peacefulness and serenity are lifting you higher into the air into the welcoming embrace of the expansive night sky. For a brief moment you understand that you exist in the space between the earth and the sky, a realm that belongs to you and is safe from anxiety. You claim this realm as yours in which to dream. This is your dreamscape, where you float towards rest and sleep. Your realm is one of peace that connects the heavens with the ground. It is yours alone to govern, to allow only positive energy and love. You roam over the tops of trees, drift across the width of lakes, and coast above others, sleeping in their warm beds.

Your entire body now is floating higher and higher in this realm as you feel such elation inside as you realize you are now gliding through all of space. You are drifting and roaming here, no longer bound by gravity. You are now soaring like a hot air balloon, ascending higher and moving towards infinity of this welcoming expands. As you float you are letting go of everything that you no longer need. You toss away unwanted negativity. You hold on to the comfort that peace grants you.

Your entire body now is floating higher and higher in this realm as you feel such elation inside as you realize you are now gliding through all of space. You are drifting and roaming here, no longer bound by gravity. You are now soaring like a hot air balloon, ascending higher and moving towards infinity of this welcoming expands. As you float you are letting go of everything you no longer need. You toss away unwanted negativity. You hold on to the comfort that peace grants you. As you become just like the pure brilliance of the stars, a beautiful shining light, you feel your spirit break free and finally you are able to float out through the entire universe. You reach out further and further into the purest wisdoms, and the most loving embraces of all of the celestial beings that surround you. They are calling you to rest, to dream, to sleep, to heal. You feel yourself realigning from within.

You feel yourself moving with tranquility and mindfulness, further and further. As you wade through the stars, you feel yourself gently feeling heavier. You understand that you are drifting towards rest.

You drift through the cosmos, feeling gravity's kind tug towards the ground. Gently you float towards the earth like a leaf falls from a tree, eager to meet its rest on the ground below. You feel completely relaxed and slipping away into a restful sleep. Before you escape into your dreams, you return to your bed where you are warm and protected. Your body softly nestles under the blankets and your head snuggles into the pillow. You notice your arms and legs still feel weightless and there is a residual warm vibration throughout, a pulsing that beseeches sleep. You happily oblige.

I am going to count down from five. When I reach one, you are going to fully embrace the peace that has engulfed you and lose yourself in sleep. You will feel yourself slipping into a calm and serene rest.

Five... You think of the night sky and its expansiveness. It melts away every remaining tension until your body and mind are relaxed. It is summoning your sleep.

Four... You feel the warmth of peace move from the top of your head and down your neck. It moves through your shoulders, radiates through your chest and stomach, and finally glazes over your legs.

Three... You feel your body become heavy and you softly sink in a little deeper to your consciousness. You are safe and protected.

Two... You feel yourself drift away, like a leaf on a still pond. You float away, quietly into the night.

One... You are now asleep, resting and at peace.

Breathe in, Breathe out. Breathe in, Breathe out. When you wake, you will be refreshed and ready to take on the day. You will be ready to conquer the stresses of your life now that you have conquered sleep.

Chapter 13 Adrenaline Addiction And High-Risk Behavior

Intent: To help warriors understand that a long-term, high-ops life tempo, along with combat experiences, leads to increased adrenaline, cortisol, and a natural high/euphoria.

Context: One of the challenges of being on deployment is that your body's homeostasis begins to acclimate to your surroundings. Thus, when in war, many unfortunately get attacked by things like RPGs or have to avoid things that are not natural in the civilian world, like IEDs. In Kandahar, we constantly got rocketed by the insurgency. The good news was that if you could hear the whizzing sound over your head, you knew it wasn't going to hit you because you could hear it. However, what you didn't know was whether there was another one on the way. And when you see the devastation that these rockets can cause to the body, ripping it to shreds, you quickly realize that you are not invincible. To mitigate this, you made sure that you hit the ground as soon as there was any indication of danger, whether that was the whizzing of rockets or an alarm indicating incoming fire. Your attention and being "on guard" was a direct result of wanting to stay alive.

This heightened sense of situational awareness and repeated exposure to stress in the AOR leaves a person in an elevated, hyped-up state, which is very similar to that of an adrenaline junkie. Yes, I said it, an adrenaline junkie. Adrenaline kept you alive when you were dodging Indirect Fire (IDF) and Direct Fire (DF). It allowed you to be sensitive to potential threats when you were risking your life on missions. It helped you cope with living in austere conditions while being away from your loved ones. It provided the energy boost necessary to keeping you effectively working 16-hour days during deployment, if not 24-hour days during combat missions. It was imperative to your survival. But you are now beginning to learn what happens to your body when it maintains elevated levels of adrenaline and cortisol over an extended period of time.

People wonder why they cannot sleep when they return home. It's because you are so used to this pace, this adrenaline, including a lack of sleep, and it's very hard to change those patterns back to baseline, especially when a person enjoys feeling very much alive. The rest of the world seems very boring once you've been "in the game." Sitting on the bench or even watching the world at its normal pace is an adrenaline junkie's nightmare. The loss of this thrilling and exciting natural drug produced by the adrenal glands is not something people want to lose. Many warriors actually deploy to a warzone repeatedly just to get the thrill of adrenaline back.

As a matter of fact, we had special ops guys who would come into the USO where I volunteered who played video games until all hours of the day and night. Instead of resting, calming down, and resetting their homeostasis, they and their buddies would stay amped up all the time on video games and power drinks. These same special ops guys actually beat the Black Ops video game within four hours of it coming out and walked out saying, "Well, that was easy."

Adrenaline Rush

The adrenaline rush is that surge of chemicals into your body that occurs under intense stress. Walter Cannon spoke of this in 1929 when he wrote about the various responses to stress: fight, flight, or freeze. Another name for adrenaline is epinephrine, and it's that intense and extremely fast chemical rush that occurs in the body when you are, for example, receiving incoming fire. It also happens when a loud noise goes off, especially when you least expect it. Controlled explosions are a little easier to take, because they usually announce them, and they are, by definition, supposed to be controlled. It's the uncontrolled explosions that really trigger our sympathetic nervous system. Just look at what happens when a car back fires near you.

Adrenaline has at least five benefits:

1. You often have a significant increase in strength (which is why you hear of a mom who lifted a car off her child who was pinned underneath);

2. Diminished feelings of pain (which is why some people can get shot and keep going);

3. Elevated senses (such as seeing, hearing, feeling, and smelling things more intensely, which is also why people are triggered by certain smells that are emotionally attached to the triggering event);

4. Significant increase in energy (which can certainly help in times when a person's life is on the line).

Unfortunately, there are at least three downsides that accompany this elevated adrenaline-junkie lifestyle.

First, it destroys the body. It's like being on methamphetamine—all the time. The body needs rest, and it has to repair itself, but anyone who has been on a natural high really dislikes having to stop. Eventually, this person not only stops but also usually crashes, which, again, can be a good thing for people with sleeping problems, but it then only trains your body to go, go, go.

I can always recognize warriors with sleeping problems because they almost always have that look of exhaustion in the morning and are drinking some type of energy-boosting beverage or any drink that contains caffeine. They often get into a bad habit of using feeling threatened at night; then they can't sleep, and then they need an upper in the morning. You can see that when the body's normal cycle is interrupted by this drug-seeking behavior, it only complicates things. For example, the body's normal repair process, when interrupted, leaves you in an anxious, jittery state. You just feel on edge, and the slightest things irritate you. The body needs rest to bring back a more normal homeostasis, but this is often interrupted twofold: first by the environment of war and second by your decisions to stay elevated. Welcome to the adrenaline-addiction world.

Second, the mind has to have time to rest to make sense of the world and what you are experiencing. Part of the problem with living at a high adrenaline level or in chronically stressful environments is that areas of your brain responsible for memory (i.e., the hippocampus) and emotional processing (i.e., the amygdala) lose nerve cells (neurons) and connections between these cells (neuronal pathways). Brain imaging studies have shown actual physical changes in size, shape, and connectivity patterns of these pivotal structures. This can be significant because this affects your ability to regulate your emotions, to encode long-term memories, and to make new memories. If you wonder why you have difficulty understanding new concepts or remembering things, it could be that you are experiencing biological changes in your brain. You knew something was wrong, but you may not have known exactly the reasons why. But it gets better, and these changes can be reversed.

Third, you don't have to like adrenaline to be exposed to chronically high levels. You may be thinking, "But I'm not an adrenaline junkie." The fact is that exposure to life-threatening situations for a prolonged period of time floods your body (and in turn, your brain) with adrenaline—whether you like it or not. Unfortunately, that's not where the story ends. It also begins to affect a stress hormone called cortisol. Cortisol is typically released in response to a threatening event or situation. Its job is to prepare the body to respond to the threat. However, in combat or disaster relief scenarios, the threat is prolonged for days, weeks, months, and, in some deployments, over a year. Our bodies are not meant to be flooded with cortisol for these extended, long periods of time. This chronic exposure causes the body to adjust to a new "normal," one in which cortisol does not ebb and flow as it does when we are in a normal, non-threatening environment. Instead, the body and brain are flooded with cortisol, leading to biological changes. These biological changes manifest themselves in symptoms that you are most likely familiar with, including memory problems, insomnia, weight gain, a weakened immune system, trouble coping, emotional outbursts, and adjustment issues.

Now let's just ask some very basic questions. Answer the following questions with a Yes or No.

Question	YES	NO
Do you have difficulty concentrating?		
Do you have difficulty remembering things?		
Do you find yourself irritable?		

Do you have difficulty sleeping?		
Have you gained weight since leaving the military?		
Do you find yourself getting sick more often than before?		

You may now be seeing the correlation between adrenaline, cortisol, and some of your problems. Much of this is biological. What does this mean for you? It means that your body is a magnificent vehicle that can adjust. And just as it adapted to develop life-saving strategies, it can be adjusted back with some of the tools and support in this workbook and through seeking out complementary treatment with a trusted, licensed therapist.

On a practical level, let's talk about what happens at night when you need the healthy systems to actually dream and not have nightmares. Nighttime is often a time when you run through the day's events and try to bring some sense of normalcy to it, but there is no "normal" in war. Trying to make sense of why people get killed, why certain decisions are being made, why we are there in the first place, missing home—you name it—is going to increase emotional responses and decrease ability to sleep. This process is interrupted mostly due to your elevated threat interpretation, which directly affects your amygdala, which, in turn, secretes more adrenaline into the bloodstream. This can then translate from normal, healthy dreams to nightmares, and this is the last thing a person wants to experience. As a matter of fact, they will do whatever they can to avoid nightmares, including purposeful sleep deprivation.

A direct correlation exists biologically between sleep deprivation and the effects of both adrenaline and cortisol. Unfortunately, through previous Stanford studies, we know that when someone goes without sleep long enough, the person can actually become psychotic. And by psychotic, we mean they can experience a break from objective reality. Do you want a combat veteran who is sleep-deprived, confused, and might become psychotic in the AOR when your life is on the line?

To be honest, you don't want an impulsive troop, especially if they have sociopathic tendencies. These are the men who take unnecessary risks that can put people's lives in danger. They are the hotheads who think they know better than everyone else. They are the first to jump up and take lead, even abandoning the mission's plans, including the commander's intent, just because they are looking for action. You can imagine this person coming back from deployment—highly anxious, sleep-deprived, angry, irritable, looking for a fight, engaging in high-risk behavior, feeling that everything is a threat, cannot get along with people, loses jobs, etc. Sound like anyone you know?

A great example of living like this is found in LTC Brad Holland. You may not know the name, but he is the guy who was infamous for living on the edge. As an adrenaline junkie, he enjoyed pushing things to the extreme. Unfortunately, Brad attempted a high-risk maneuver that pushed his B-52 bomber beyond the limits of its capacity to fly. In preparation for an air show, he lost airspeed in a high-banking maneuver, which created an unrecoverable crash and subsequent explosion. The event, caught on camera, is often used to illustrate how high-risk behavior can cost people their lives. His copilot, the only guy who would copilot with him, and two other crew members died that day.

Coming Home

If any of these symptoms sound familiar to you, you may be an adrenaline junkie. Let's be clear: it has its benefits, but it also has its pitfalls. People often talk about going to substance abuse counseling, but when was the last time you ever heard of a debriefing on being an adrenaline addict? Let's take a little test to see how you would rate.

Adrenaline Addiction Test

Question	YES	NO
I drink power drinks or coffee or take stimulants to maintain energy.		

I seek out exciting, outdoor, high-risk behavior to keep me happy.		
I feel anxious/jittery.		
I wait until the last minute to do things and then rush to get them done.		
I feel that the rest of the world is boring.		
Others tell me that I overreact to situations, or I can sense they want to tell me but won't.		
I am always in the "on" position; "off" is best illustrated by exhaustion.		
I am easily startled by things.		
I find that when I'm not in control, things really bother me.		

I hardly ever feel a sense of calm, relaxation, or peace.		
I believe that losing is not an option and winning is correlated to effort; others don't try hard enough, and they easily frustrate me.		
I walk around a lot, and taking tests is a waste of my time.		
I am easily agitated by other people's driving habits.		
Being on time is not an option because I'm hardly ever on time.		
I am a firm believer that others simply want an easy life; they have no idea how vulnerable they are, and they would be easily killed by a terrorist.		

Finances are always a challenge because I spend money as soon as I get it.		
Focus and concentration are great as long as I'm being asked to focus on something I'm excited about; if not, you have my attention for about five minutes, and then I'm off in my head.		
Go, go, go is a motto; hurry up and wait is a stupid concept.		
When people are talking, I've already tuned them out.		
I sometimes have pressured speech because I have so much to say that I can't even get out what my brain is thinking.		
Racing thoughts occur at night when I'm trying to go to bed.		
I wonder if people think I'm crazy.		

Motorcycles, rock climbing, skydiving, and bungee jumping are things I would do in a heartbeat.		
My legs are jumping while taking this test.		
I have a very high sex drive.		
These are stupid questions; get on with it.		

Although this is not a standardized test, let's see how you did. Add up your yes answers and see the scoring chart below.

Scoring key

- 1–5: minimal adrenaline

- 6–10: moderate adrenaline

- 11 or higher: Let's just not go there, as your irritability may surface.

Consequences

Unfortunately, people do not often change their behavior until consequences force them to. For example, you may not have sought treatment had it not been for loved ones or friends who basically indicated you needed help. They may not have known what to do, but they did know that something was wrong. Unfortunately, too many times we are thrown into a situation where we are forced to change because of consequences, which can be due to legal issues, marital/relationship issues, suicidal/homicidal ideation, mental health challenges, or a series of other reasons. Whatever the reason, we are glad you are reading this workbook.

The best way to change the addiction to adrenaline is to:

- First, realize what it is doing to your body. You have to be convinced that adrenaline and high-risk behavior are not good for you. Adrenaline causes heart palpitations, tachycardia (racing heart), arrhythmia (irregular heart beat), anxiety, panic attacks, headaches, tremors, hypertension, strokes, heart attacks, kidney damage, and acute pulmonary edema. None of these symptoms are enjoyable to live with, and over a long period of time, some can actually kill you. Isn't it interesting that, once again, the same thing that kept you alive in a theater may eventually kill you if not treated properly?

Between 5-10% of all visits to U.S. Emergency Departments are patients feeling as if they are having a heart attack. After thorough evaluation, they find out their heart is fine and that the effects of adrenaline are causing the anxiety/panic attacks. You won't die, but you have to learn how to control your anxiety.

Growing up, I was taught the art of moderation. The idea is that a person who is addicted to adrenaline is, unfortunately, off the chart regarding moderation. The consequences of this high adrenaline create many of the same symptoms we are trying to mitigate.

- Second, adrenaline affects memory consolidation. Adrenaline affects retrograde (past) memories to where they consolidate at a higher rate. During highly emotionally, stressful times, adrenaline creates a strong bond between intense emotional states, such as fear and memory consolidation. This is exactly why people with PTS(D) often remember their negative experiences in vivid detail. It is also common for people to try to use avoidance to not remember, but their own biology makes it almost impossible. For most of us, it doesn't take much, such as a particular smell or sound, to trigger us into a reflective moment called a flashback. We certainly don't teach ourselves to do this; it is a biological response that the brain has created. Remember that the brain's intent is to keep you alive, and it did; otherwise, you wouldn't be reading this. However, you are also no longer in a war zone, and it's time to get you back.

- Third, we need to retrain your brain that not everything is a threat. Since we were taught risk assessment, this is where we actually need to use it. What is important at this juncture is to understand that there is a clear biological reason why you interpret situations and people as a threat, even if they have no ill intent. This topic is so vital that we wrote a complete module to address it. "Module IX: Possibility vs. Probability" specifically focuses on threat assessment and risk mitigation.

- Fourth, we will never forget. I can only speculate that Adam and Eve had nightmares after Cain killed Abel. Do you think for one second that they could ever forget what happened? NO! I'm sure they even blamed themselves and their parenting skills. Instead, we have to find a way to resolve our grief/loss and other issues, which is why we created the following modules: moral injury, survival guilt, and perspective.

- Fifth, increasing one's resiliency factor and finding resolution is key. Let me explain it this way. When Chris Kyle, the highly decorated American sniper, was asked if he ever had regrets for killing so many people, he could have said, "Well, I was brought up in church and taught to not kill. I also believe in the Ten Commandments. So, yes, these memories haunt me, and I can never get away from them. I see the faces of the people I killed, and at night I cannot forget them. I feel as if I will be in hell for what I did. I do not deserve forgiveness." But that is not what he said. He had resolved the killings in his mind, and, although paraphrased, his comment sounded something like this: "I only regret that I could not have killed more of our enemies so that more of our guys could have lived." Now that is a person who has resolved in his mind a potential internal conflict. In psychological terms, he is ego-syntonic with his thoughts, because, in the end, he was protecting our men by his actions. What our intent will be is to help you become ego-syntonic with your thoughts and actions to the point of resiliency and resolution.

Chapter 14 Deep Sleep Techniques

Meditation To Overcome Insomnia

Whether you find it difficult to sleep at night as a result of stress, tiredness, work or several other factors, or you find your sleep unsatisfactory, you might be suffering from insomnia. Insomnia is commonly called difficulty falling asleep, or staying awake, and there two types of insomnia.

Acute insomnia is mostly caused as a result of lifestyle, or circumstances. A security officer on night duty will find it difficult to fall asleep on duty, likewise a first-time dad may find it difficult to fall asleep thinking of his precious wife in labor.

While, chronic insomnia is a complicated type of insomnia. There is no known underlying cause, yet the individual finds it difficult to either fall asleep, or sleep at night for long hours. Such person may also experience disrupted sleep, for more than 3 times a week.

Experiencing insomnia regularly causes mood disturbances, fatigue, stress and difficulty concentrating. Although, insomnia can be caused by factors like anxiety, work related stress, lifestyle, and sicknesses. However, the approach to overcome insomnia is not easy for some persons, yet there is one possible way to overcome not just insomnia but enjoy a long, satisfactory sleep for the rest of your life.

How Does Meditation Cure Insomnia

Meditation is a relaxation technique worth trying, which can help improve your sleep, make you fall asleep easily and also make your sleep satisfactory, such that you wake up feeling refreshed. Meditation harmonizes the mind and body, and also influences the brain and the way it functions. The effect of meditation on your mind and body is that you become calm, and relaxed afterwards.

Effect of Meditation on Insomnia

During meditation, the mind is focused on one thing, which prevents the mind from wandering. Your mind and thoughts are brought to the now moment during meditation. Hence, anxiety disappears and it becomes easier to fall asleep.

During the meditation, your mind and body are been connected to each other, and they both become relaxed and calm, which helps you sleep as soon as you get in bed.

Furthermore, meditation helps boost the hormone called melatonin that regulates the sleep and wake cycle. Without stress, the melatonin level is usually at its peak at night to ensure you get a sound, and restful sleep. However, the presence of stress among other factors that causes insomnia, the melatonin level drastically reduces, thereby insomnia occurs. With meditation, the melatonin level increases because stress has been reduced, and the body is in a relaxed state.

Meditation Techniques for Insomnia

If you want to experience an undisrupted sleep, an intense meditation must be done frequently. There are different techniques of meditating for insomnia and understanding process help us to get started immediately.

- Cognitive shuffling

Cognitive shuffling is a simple meditation technique that can be done alone. It is simply a do-it-yourself technique that shuffles your thoughts to sleep. Here is how cognitive shuffling works, when you lie on your bed, your mind is likely to be filled with different thoughts from your daily activities. You can be worried, and anxious about your bills, relationship, the next day activities, such that you find it difficult to fall asleep. The effect of this shuffling on the brain is it tricks the mind to get into a dreaming state.

Tips to Practice Cognitive Shuffling

- Firstly, getting in bed is important

- Right there on your bed, avoid focusing your concerns. Let your deadline be, the bills, the complicated issue at work. Let it all be.

- Now that your mind is free from your fears and worries, create a new engagement like imagining objects, places, names or movies to meditate on. You can imagine different things, like a teddy bear, a fish, a dog, the sky, the rainbow, or the ocean. Note that, the items you are imagining should not be threatening or scary. For instance, instead of imagining an ocean because you have the fear of water, you can imagine the rainbow or the sky with beautiful stars.

- Ensure your eyes are closed before you begin the cognitive shuffling process.

- Process should be repeated if you are still awake, until you run out of words.

- Sa Ta Na Ma (Mantra)

Sa Ta Na Ma is a powerful meditation technique that works on the brain and its functions to reduce risk of depression and other mental illness. It is a mantra that is usually recited in 3 voices; the singing voice which stands for the action voice.

The whispered voice which stands for your inner voice, and

The silent voice is known as your spirit's voice.

SA TA NA MA chant describes the evolutionary aspect of the universe. Each word in the chant has a meaning.

SA means the beginning.

TA means existence and creativeness

NA means death or the end of life

MA means rebirth

The effect of this mantra is displayed by a balance in emotions, and a settled mind.

Practical steps to Sa Ta Na Ma

-       Find a comfortable position. You can sit down or lie down.

-       Decide on how many minutes you want to recite the mantra.

-       Breathe in and out through your nose and mouth and ensure you sigh after this breathing exercise is heard.

-       Close your eyes properly, and place your hands either on your lap, or knee. Make sure your palm is facing up.

-       Begin chanting slowly, and press the thumb of your hands, with your four fingers. Count your fingers each starting from the thumb to recite the mantra.

-       Keep reciting the chant as a calm and slow pace

During recitation, you have to follow the principles of the mantra.

When you mention SA, you count from your index to your thumb

You count from your middle finger to your thumb when you sing TA

You count from your ring finder to thumb when you recite NA

And final you should count from your pinky finger to the thumb when you mention MA.

-       Still in that position, sing SA TA NA MA in a loud voice, your voice should be audible, and ensure you move each of your fingers with each sound. The more you sing, the more you feel relaxed and energetic. However, your soul and spirit should feel relaxed and enjoy the sensation which is moving through your body and mind.

- When you feel relaxed, shift your focus and start singing in a whisper voice. At this point, energy is flowing through the body, waist, and knee.

- Next, be focused on silence. Continue counting your fingers and silently repeat the mantra to yourself.

- After singing the mantra completely, breathe in and breathe out with your arms wide open, and lift the hand above your head. Release your hands down, and exhale again. Repeat process until you feel refreshed or drowsy.

What to Expect When Meditating To Fall Asleep

Your expectations when meditating to fall asleep is most likely to have a sound and deep sleep at night, except you are uncertain about the benefits of meditation. Meditation for sleep is similar to other kind of meditation; however, the approach to each of these meditations is what matters.

When meditating, your meditation technique determines what you will have to do. Albeit, you can start preparing for your meditation exercise, by breathing in and out, lying flat on your back. If you are having a guided meditation, all you need to do is follow the instructions instead of been worried about what to do and what not to do.

Furthermore, all you should when meditating to fall asleep is sleep, but try to avoid any form of distractions.

How to Meditate Before Sleep

There are two ways you can meditate before going to bed, it can be a mindful meditation where you pay more attention to your body and mind, and also having a guided meditation where someone leads you through the process of meditation.

Mindfulness meditation can be done alone, in your own room house and house. While guided meditation is a very easy meditation, it is just for you to follow and listen to instructions from a guide.

Guided Meditation Tips For Insomnia

Guided meditation is the form of meditation you engage in with the help of a tutor, or instructor. Ensure that you will not be disturbed, during the course of this meditation.

-       Lay down on your back, preferably on your bed or mat. Make sure you are comfortable on whatever you are lying on.

-       Close your eyes and prepare your mind for the meditation you are about to engage in.

-       Breathe in and out, ensure that your breathing out is audible such that it looks like you breathing out heavily. Make your body feel the heaviness, after which your body will be relaxed.

-     Pay more attention to your breathing, and you feel easiness. A natural breathing process.

-     At this point, you will feel your body is relaxed. Feel the way your breath travels through your lungs, and hold your breath. As this is happening, you will begin to feel relaxation in your body.

-     You can begin to breathe normally right now, and as you breathe you feel your muscles, joints, and back relaxed.

-     Pay more attention to your stomach area right now, where your abdominal muscles are present. Tighten the muscles in your abdomen, and hold your breath for 10 seconds and release your muscles. During this release, feel the difference the tightness of your abdominal muscle and the relaxation of these muscles.

-     Repeat the above process 5 times.

-     Breathe in and out, tighten your abdomen and release it to relaxation.

Feet

-     Divert your attention to your feet, and make them relaxed. The relaxation should be from your toes to your ankles.

Tighten your toes and feet, and feel them become heavy and relaxed.

-      Focus on your nails, feel them relaxed and let go.

-      Pay attention to your thigh area, and feel them relaxed.

-      Again, focus on your waist, lower and upper back, joints and feel them relaxed. You will feel the feel heavy, and very relaxed

Upper limbs

-      At this point, focus your attention on your arms. Feel them heavy and relaxed.

-      Get a sense of how heavy your arm is, and feel the relaxation shift to your elbow, wrist, and fingers become very relaxed.

Face, neck and facial muscles

-      Shift your focus to your facial muscles, neck and face.

-      Every muscle in your face, your cheeks and chin becomes relaxed, and your entire body is now relaxed.

A deeper meditation for the abdomen

-      Locate your center, which is your abdominal region. Imagine there is a bowl on your abdomen. Slowly see the bowl rolling over your abdomen area, and it relaxes every muscle the bowl rolls in contact with.

- The bowl now moves slowly from your abdomen area to your right hip carefully and softly massaging the muscles of the hips it comes in contact to.

- Massaging back and forth all the muscles in your abdomen.

- The ball continues to roll over to your knee, and around your knee. You can feel the tension on your navel melting away. Roll the ball slowly to your toe, and over to your toes, from your small toes to the big toes.

Every part of your body this ball comes in contact with feel the part of your body relaxing.

- Now feel the ball begins to roll upwards away from your toes again. Massaging and reducing tension around your toes, knees, ankles and rolls over to your center, your abdominal area.

- Again, this balls rolls to your left thigh, and your knee, massaging both the back and front of your knee.

With your ball you move this ball to wherever you choose, and how long you want it to be.

- With this ball, massage your knee, and ankle and toes. This ball touches every muscle in your toes, it gently massages them and at this point, you feel your muscle relax.

- Feel the ball roll back up your leg, your knee and thigh muscle and arriving back at your center.

- Shift the focus of the ball to the base of your spinal cord. Allow the ball rest there for 5 seconds, and allow it move up your spine, and near your heart. At this point, you can feel the ball massaging the internal organs in your body. The ball massages the heart, and you feel relaxed.

- The ball rolls to your throat area, and the back of your neck area. You feel your neck area relaxing after the ball massages it. You feel tension reducing around your neck area.

- The ball travels down your arm, and to your wrist. The ball gently massages your wrist, and fingers.

- You feel the ball roll up your arm, to your shoulder and neck. It travels down to your elbow, forearm, and wrist and into the palm of your hands.

- Allow the ball gently massage your palm, and fingers. The ball moves up your arm, shoulder and face and as it reaches up in your face, the ball splits into a hundred tiny balls. You feel them travel around your face, to your eyes, eyebrow, cheeks, chin, teeth, tongue and teeth.

- You feel the ball massaging your face and every part of your face. At this point, you should enjoy this facial massage.

- I want you to imagine as you are lying down the ceiling of your house. Youreyes is still closed, so imagine the ceiling of your room opening itself up, and the roof also opens itself open.

- Still looking at this opening, you will see the beautiful white sky. The sky is clear, bright, and the moon is out and also full, filled with stars. This is a magical peaceful night. You are alone, safe in the beautiful part of your house.

- Watch the twinkling and beautiful little stars, looking down on you and you are enjoying the peace of the night.

- You look again at the stars again, the little ones that are thousands of miles away are not shining so beautiful like the big star closer to you, that is looking at you directly from the sky.

- You are looking deep into galaxy, beyond time, you see a million other stars waiting for you and shining at you.

- Take a deep breath. breathe in a rich air from the infinite and beautiful galaxy filled with stars.

- Feel yourself been a part of these stars, there is no separation between you and them. Feel you are already a part of this wonderful galaxy.

- As you experience this, you become a shooting star, shining across the galaxy like others.

-       Slowly you begin to fade into the sky, into the unending space and galaxy.

-       You are living in the wonders of this space, where there is neither time, past or future. You feel you are the stars, the moon, and you occupy the pace between the planets.

-       You are floating off slowly, as you travel across this universe; you feel your body wants to drift away. You feel peace, wholeness, and love.

-       When you are ready, and feel relaxed, you can let go of the galaxy. When you drift off, you will drift into a peaceful and wonderful sleep.

Guided Meditation For Insomnia In Pregnant Women

Meditation for pregnant women can seem difficult; however, the need to be relaxed is very important, to reduce tension, and frustration. Below are some tips to help you meditate as a pregnant woman.

-       Pick a comfortable position, you can lie on your back, or sit upright. Ensure you feel comfortable.

-       Take a deep breath, and take another deep breath for your baby.

- You are aware of your strong, beautiful and shaped body. You are aware of your baby and how beautiful the baby is.

- Ensure that you feel and observe the sensation that comes as you breathe in and out. As you are breathing in, your body is getting relaxed, and tension is reduced.

- Remember that you are pregnant and meditation can be difficult as this stage; however, take your time to be patient while meditating. Try to avoid every form of distraction around you.

- Find a quiet place to be alone for 10 – 15 minutes. Sit in an upright position, and make sure you are comfortable.

- If you are lying in bed, focus your attention on the bed, by imagining that you are sinking into bed. And if you are sitting, create an imagination of your body in contact with your mattress, and also sinking into it.

- Begin to sense what it feels like to sink into your bed. Notice if you feel lighter, or heavy. Then begin awareness on your body to observe any tension and tightness around your body, from your head to toe.

- Focus your attention on any part of your body you desire, and become aware of the part of the body. Breathe in and out. Get a picture of that part, feel the tension melting away and tightness reducing.

- You can scan your body mes in 5 minutes. During this scan, observe and note places that are relaxed or still tight.

- Practice more breathing pattern here. Breathe in and breathe out, for the first 2 minutes, observe your breathing pattern, and focus on your breathing, without a motive to change it. You may start to notice that your breathing becomes slower on its own. You may also notice the way your body moves when you breathe. If your chest rises more than your belly does, it means your breathing is shallow.

- However, a shallow breathing is just a pattern that shows our state of relaxation. If you are relaxed, your belly will rise more than your chest.

- Place your hands on your bell, and feel your baby.

- Observe the movements in your belly with your hands,

- Think about your day, in a structured way. Look back at every activity you did during the day. Remember when your baby kicked, when you went to see the doctor, when you had a funny and interesting conversation with your friends. Be patient to watch these moments as your brain play them back for you. These flashbacks may seem long or short, it all depends on how your day went. Keep enjoying this flashback, focus your mind on it and avoid been distracted and watch as these events unfold to the present moment.

- Shift your focus back to your baby. Place your attention on your feet, toes and tell them to switch off. You can literally say the word 'switch off' out so that you feel you have told your body parts they are not needed until the next day.

- Repeat exercise and inform your upper limbs, your arms, hands, wrist and fingers to switch off.

- Repeat your breathing exercise again.

- Place your hands on your belly, and say the following words

You are a miracle, and not a trouble.

You will allow me have a restful night

You will be patient with me till I am awake.

You are healthy and strong."

- After saying those words, breathe in and out gain for yourself and your baby.

- Imagine that your baby is falling asleep. Pay more attention on how your baby looks and the way your baby breathes.

- At this point, I believe you should be asleep. If you are not yet asleep, you can repeat exercise and allow your mind get relaxed.

Guided Meditation For Insomnia In Children

Guided meditation is a type of meditation, where there is an instructor. Little children do not have to that the knowledge to meditate on their own, so their parents can guide them into this meditation using the following.

-      Welcome to your happy moment. We will start an adventure right now.

-      Make sure you are lying down properly, on your bed, if you feel pain because of the way you lie down, let your parent or guardian know.

-      Close your eyes properly and begin to imagine things the sun, how it is so clear and shining. Do not open your eyes.

-      Start releasing your body, and everything you are thinking of. So, tighten your muscles, your arms and legs, for a few seconds.

-      Let your arms get released, with your legs too. Enjoy the relaxation now, as your muscles are released

-      Try the process again, tighten your arms and legs and release them later.

-      Start breathing in and breathing out. Make sure you hear the sound that comes out when you breathe in and out.

- Release the air you have breathed in from your lungs, and breathe out.

- Repeat the breathing exercise, breathe in and out and relaxed.

- Now, imagine yourself in a beautiful and dark garden like the wonderland. This wonderland is dark, because it is night.

- You feel the ground is so soft that you feel like sinking into it.

- You feel a gentle and soft breeze on your face and body. The wonderland is so cool and beautiful; you don't want to leave there.

- At this point, you see your body becoming relaxed.

- You look up, and set the beautiful sun set, and the birds flying around in the wonderland.

- You continue walking; you look at the beautiful trees, with fruits on it.

- You keep walking until you see a colorful tent in front of you. The tent is the color of the rainbow. It is so beautiful; you walk into the tent.

- As you go into the tent, you see how beautiful it is. It has a beautiful sofa with the rainbow color, the wall of the tent has the pictures of all your heroes, and you like the way the tent is.

-      The tents has different rooms, the living room has a Television set with your favorite cartoon, the kitchen has the pictures of your favorite food, the room has big soft bed, you feel the softness as you touch it, and there is a big pool where you can swim before the kitchen.

-      Keep walking around to see how beautiful this tent is.

-      Now, you are done looking around this magical tent in your wonderland. You walk out of the tent, and you see another beautiful garden that surrounds the tent.

-      This garden is so beautiful. You are walking around and you see a table with two chairs, a jug of juice, and two glass cups.

-      You drink a glass of juice, and look around to see if there is anyone around you.

-      You then see someone walking towards you; the person is smiling at you. The person is happy, and keeps smiling at you.

-      You offer the person a glass of juice, the person receives it happily and drinks.

-      You show this person around your magical tent.

-      Did you have a beautiful talk with your new friend?

-    You hug your visitor softly, and you watch the person go away.

-    You breathe in and out and you feel happy and relaxed right now.

-    At this point you are feeling sleepy, so you walk back into the tent and walk into your room to lie on your soft and rainbow color bed.

-    You tuck yourself into your bed, and place your head on the soft pillow.

-    You feel your body sinking into your bed. Your arms are feeling relaxed, and your hips to your toes are feeling relaxed.

-    There is a window in your room, so you lie on your side to watch the beautiful dark sky and you also see the big shining star in the center of the sky.

-    You smile and feel happy; you tell yourself you are a big shining star.

-    You look at the other shining stars; they look beautiful just for you.

-    You see them moving together fast; you wonder where they are going. They are going to the galaxy, so you decide to join them.

-	You see yourself floating into the dark clouds, and far beyond the clouds, you see more stars.

-	You are happy now, and very sleepy.

-	You begin to drift away. You are getting sleepier, so you return to your soft bed.

-	You cannot open our eyes now, because you are already deep into your sleep.

-	You mind and body is now relaxed and quiet.

-	At this point, you are fast asleep.

Conclusion

I want to thank you once again for purchasing this book.

If you want to improve your focus, live a stress-free life, and manage your anxiety, then follow the simple exercises on guided meditation given in this book.

The exercises mentioned in this book will help you live a happier life and enable you to let go of all the unnecessary worries in your life so that you can concentrate on the things that matter to you. It hardly takes ten minutes to go through each of these guided meditation exercises. All that you need to do is find a comfortable spot for yourself, turn off all distractions, and listen to the meditation exercises. Within no time, you will be able to see a positive change in your life.

Repeat these meditations as needed. The more that you practice them, the easier it will be to find valuable healing benefits within them. As with all meditations, ensure that you never do them while operating a vehicle as you could fall asleep. Also, ensure that you find a quiet space free of any distractions.

After you have practiced meditation a few times, you could try to do it somewhere else, such as on an airplane or traveling when you are not the one who is in charge of moving the vehicle.

It could help you relax in the right settings, but you have to get used to what you might do after these meditative practices. The more that you practice them, the easier it will be for your mind to click into this place when necessary.

Check out the other meditation books in the series to find something valuable based on your specific needs. Keep an open mind and allow healing into your life whenever possible.

www.ingramcontent.com/pod-product-compliance
Lightning Source LLC
Chambersburg PA
CBHW070704250726
48662CB00001B/243